D1807836

CONTENTS

Introduction

This guide provides an overview of the best-known alternative cancer treatments. It is not an exhaustive list but represents the alternative treatments that are the most widely used by people with cancer, which have stood the test of time and for which there is the most evidence. All the information given is based on the available knowledge at the point of writing and is given in good faith to help lighten the task of those with cancer who urgently need to find helpful information in order to explore their treatment options.

It is hoped that the many alternative cancer treatments described in this guide will give you positive choices in making your own treatment plan. However, you may be left feeling that you need help to decide which alternative treatments are right for you.

There are three good sources of help available to you.

- Integrated or holistic cancer doctors, who specialise in the integration of alternative, complementary, nutritional, self help and psycho-spiritual support for the healing of cancer.

- Alternative cancer doctors, who specialise in alternative cancer medicine for the treatment of cancer.

- Cancer Options, a service established by a cancer nurse that offers a review of the alternative treatment options presented by different doctors and clinics worldwide.

Contact points for all of these sources of help are to be found in the Resource Guide at the back of this book.

This guide does not cover the use of healthy eating and juicing for combating cancer, nor self-help mind-body approaches, as these are covered in the Health Creation Programme in the Cancer Lifeline Kit, from which this guide comes.

The information given about each alternative cancer treatment is classified under the seven headings with references to the source material listed at the end of this guide.

Background including the origins of the remedy where known.

Uses and dosage describing the primary uses of the substance and typical dosage range.

How to use indicating if the treatment can be bought and self-administered by an individual or whether it must be prescribed and administered by doctors or nurses in a medical setting. Also if is safe to use alongside conventional treatment.

Drug interactions and special precautions highlighting any specific cautions and information to be aware of when using the treatment.

Mechanism of action is described if known or, alternatively, the theory upon which the use of the treatment is given.

Level of evidence in which the evidence supporting the use of the treatment is classified.

• Randomised controlled trial – described as the 'gold standard' of high-quality scientific research. In this type of study subjects have been matched with controls that do not get the treatment. Neither the patients nor the doctors know who is getting the active treatment. This methodology eliminates bias and placebo effects from the results, so that the effectiveness of the treatment can be assessed objectively.

• Pure science – where a treatment has been tested in the laboratory to establish the active constituent and the probable mechanism of action.

• Case study – where a series of patients who have taken a treatment have been studied by doctors and a clinical impression has been gathered over time as to the value of the treatment.

• Anecdotal evidence – where the benefits of a treatment are described and passed on from patient to patient on the basis of their personal experience.

• Traditional treatment – where the approach is part of an ancient system of treatment that has been passed down by practitioners from generation to generation.

• Epidemiological – where the disease patterns in populations are studied.

Source and price indicating where the treatment can be obtained and the approximate cost at the time of printing this guide.

The reason many alternative cancer treatments have not yet become mainstream, despite the evidence for their benefits, may have may have much to do with political control over the cancer medicine 'market'. The politics of cancer are believed by many to have an overriding influence on the direction of cancer science, what we are led to think and believe about cancer and what you can expect to be offered as treatment options. The facts behind this controversy are beyond the scope of this book, however if you are interested in making your own judgement on this matter there are numerous agencies to refer to. Two of the liveliest and most controversial sources of information and opinion on this subject come from Dr Samuel Epstein in his book 'The Politics of Cancer' and Dr Ralph Moss in his book 'The Cancer Industry: Unravelling the Politics' (see ref 14).

Using alternative cancer treatments

Alternative cancer treatments are used singly in some cases and in combination in others. They ideally form part of an integrated treatment approach that includes nutrition, vitamin and mineral supplementation as well as self-help mind-body techniques, psychological and spiritual support, energy treatments, and often conventional medicine too.

The exact combination of therapies and treatments depends entirely on the individual and their unique circumstances, needs and preferences. Whilst it is perfectly safe for individuals to initiate the use of many of these treatments themselves, the use of more complex regimes should be supervised by a holistic doctor or alternative cancer clinic. It is also wise to take holistic medical advice prior to starting these treatments, particularly while having chemotherapy or radiotherapy, or if you are pregnant or on other medication. Any side-effects of treatment should be discussed immediately with your holistic doctor.

Using this guide

The guide is intended to provide you with an awareness of some of the alternative approaches that are available to fight cancer so that you may have informed discussions about your options with your holistic, alternative or conventional medical team.

The information given does not imply an endorsement of any particular alternative cancer treatment on the part of the authors, and the authors assume no medical responsibility for anyone who chooses to initiate treatment themselves without the supervision of a holistic/alternative cancer doctor or clinic. The Resource Directory at the end of this guide provides information on useful books, websites, alternative cancer doctors, holistic cancer doctors and clinics, the Cancer Options service, and suppliers of all of the treatments and services mentioned.

Continuing to build the picture

If you have any other useful information or evidence relating to these alternative cancer treatments we would be very interested to hear from you, as this is a living document that will be updated when new information becomes available. We would also like to know if you think we have omitted any important alternative cancer treatment.

1 Anti-cancer nutrients

Diet and nutrition have been shown in numerous scientific studies to play a key role in the prevention and treatment of cancer. A healthy diet with vitamin and mineral supplementation is an essential part of any anti-cancer regime. The following section highlights some specific nutritional supplements that have been acknowledged as useful in helping to maintain optimum nutrition, immune system functioning and tissue healing.

Antioxidant formulations

Background

In recent years antioxidant vitamins, minerals and plant extracts have been increasingly highlighted as playing an important role in protecting the cell's genetic material and membranes from free-radical damage, thus preserving normal cell reproduction and all-round functioning. They are now considered to be a vital element of all holistic cancer treatment and prevention plans.

The antioxidant formulation is used to help the body reduce free-radical damage and strengthen the immune system. Dosage varies according to patient's condition.

A baseline level of antioxidants for the first year post diagnosis of cancer.

Vitamin C	food state – 500 mg three times per day
	as calcium ascorbate – 1 gram three times per day
Beta-carotene	food state – 13.5 mg daily

Please note This is equivalent to 1.5 pints (3 litres) of carrot juice. Reduce your dose of beta-carotene appropriately depending on the amount of juice being taken each day.

Vitamin E	food state – 400 IU daily
Vitamin B	food state complex – 50 mg daily
Selenium	200 micrograms daily
Zinc	as elemental zinc – 15 mg daily
	as zinc orotate – 100 mg daily
	as zinc citrate – 50 mg daily

Please note Doses of zinc should be reduced to a third of these levels three months after the end of treatment to prevent excess accumulation of zinc in the tissues. Taken during treatment, zinc helps to promote tissue healing greatly.

How to use

Antioxidant formulations are usually taken orally in tablet form and may be self-administered. It is desirable to take antioxidants alongside conventional treatments, as they enhance their effectiveness. Do not take antioxidants on the day of chemotherapy treatment, as this may weaken the effect of the chemotherapy.

In alternative cancer clinics antioxidant vitamins and minerals are also given intravenously in mega doses, almost like a form of natural chemotherapy for tumour destruction. The most effective is high-dose vitamin C. The other commonly used vitamin is B17 or laetrile, which contains cyanide that helps to cause tumour destruction (see page 24).

Mechanism of action

A free radical is an unstable molecule with an unpaired electron that steals an electron from another molecule and in doing so produces harmful effects. Free radicals are produced in the body by external harmful influences such as radiation, frying and barbecuing food, and environmental pollution; and by internal processes, as a by-product of metabolism. Free radicals are also produced during radiation and chemotherapy. To protect the body against these free radicals it is important that the body has sufficient quantities of antioxidants.

An antioxidant is a natural biochemical substance that protects living cells against damage from harmful free radicals. If unblocked or left uncontrolled, oxidation can lead to cellular ageing, degeneration, allergies, arthritis, heart disease, cancer and other illnesses. Antioxidants in the body react readily with free radicals and neutralise them before they can damage the body.

Antioxidant nutrients include vitamins A, C and E, beta-carotene, selenium, zinc, coenzyme Q10, pycnogenol (grape seed extract), L-glutahione, superoxide dismutase and bioflavonoids. When antioxidants are taken in combination, the effect is stronger than when they are used individually.

The amount of antioxidants in the system makes the critical difference between a normal functioning immune system and the initiation of a potential cancer process. When free-radical production exceeds the ability of the immune system's neutralising mechanisms, progressive cellular damage can begin. When this damage becomes chronic, the next step is chronic or serious degenerative disease, including cancer.

Free radicals are particularly dangerous as they have a tendency to attack and destroy fragile membranes surrounding cells, thus making the body more vulnerable to various cancer initiators and promoters. In addition, free radicals themselves may interact with cellular DNA, causing mutations that can lead to cancer formation.[1]

Although antioxidants are available naturally in foods, to offset intense free-radical activity, people often need to enhance the process with antioxidant supplements, especially if their diet is, or has been, nutritionally inadequate for some time. Although many antioxidants such as vitamin C can neutralise free radicals, on doing so, the antioxidant become inert and loses its ability to neutralise further free radicals. Newer 'cascading' antioxidants retain their neutralising ability and are therefore more potent than the antioxidant vitamins.

Level of evidence

The importance of antioxidants to the optimum functioning of bodily systems such as the immune systems has been studied through a variety of pure science and laboratory studies. There are more than 10,000 peer reviewed studies of the role of anti-oxidants in cancer prevention and treatment, which range through epidemiological, pure science and prospective randomised controlled trials.

In China a prospective trial in which 50,000 Chinese were given selenium, vitamin E, beta-carotene and zinc at levels on page 8 showed a 13.5% decrease in deaths from cancer of all types after 5 years.

Source and price

High quality 'Food State' vitamins and minerals that are highly bio-available to the body are made by Nature's Own.

The cost of a month's supply at the levels on page 8 is £58.16.

Neways International have developed a product called Cascading Revenol that contains 23 antioxidants in a regenerative formulation that has a sustained release delivery system to enhance the body's ability to neutralise damaging free-radicals.

Cascading Revenol's formulation regenerates the antioxidant molecules after they have exerted their effect to enable them to neutralise multiple free radicals. Therefore instead of only one free radical being destroyed per antioxidant molecule, each molecule is continuously able to repeat the process of neutralising free radicals.

The formulation combines water-soluble white pine bark (pycnogenol) and oil-soluble grape seed extract, together with turmeric extract (curcuminoids). Key minerals and trace elements such as zinc, copper and selenium are complexed with amino acids to promote absorption through the intestinal tract. Vitamin C is supplied in an esterfied form that enhances its power and residual retention in the body for up to three days.

Other ingredients include decaffeinated green tea extract, inositol, coenzyme Q10, vitamin E, carotenoid complex, ellagic acid, astaxanthin, resveratrol, glutathione, rosemary officinalis extract, citrus bioflavonoid complex, quercitin, taurine, n-acetyl cysteine and potassium sulphate. This combination of potent antioxidants makes it one of the most effective antioxidant products that is available.

Cascading Revenol is taken orally as capsules and may be self-administered. It costs £65.80 for a month's supply.

Intravenous antioxidant therapy is available from the alternative doctors and clinics listed in the Resource Directory. The cost is available upon enquiry.

Multi-mineral formulations

Background

Numerous studies have shown the importance of minerals for regulating many of the physiological processes in the body and in protecting the body from cancer. In particular selenium, zinc, copper, chromium and manganese have been identified as playing important roles in cancer prevention because of their antioxidant role, their role in maintaining the correct functioning of the immune system and for enhanced tissue healing.

Uses and dosage

Multi-minerals are used to help provide the body with the appropriate level of minerals for optimum functioning and to strengthen the immune and tissue systems. Dosage varies according to the patient's condition and the preparation used.

How to use

Multi-minerals are usually taken orally and may be self-administered. In alternative cancer clinics they may be given by doctors as part of an intravenous drip treatment with appropriate antioxidant vitamins.

Mechanism of action

Selenium has key effects on DNA metabolism, cell membrane integrity and optimal functioning of both the liver and pancreas. As such it can interfere with both the initiation and promotion phases of cancer development. Glutathione peroxidase protects tissues against free radical damage and its anti-cancer effects are greatly dependent on the availability of selenium.[2]

Like selenium, zinc supports many aspects of the immune system and its deficiency can potentially make the body more vulnerable to certain cancers. Zinc is necessary for the free radical quenching activity of superoxidase dismutase (SOD), a powerful antioxidant that breaks down the free radical superoxide to form hydrogen peroxide. A deficiency of zinc can lead to depressed activity of NK cells and of the other white blood cells.[3]

Copper is also essential to proper functioning of a wide range of immune cells types, including antibody forming cells, T helper cells and macrophages, all of which help defend the body against cancer.[4] Copper functions as a cofactor for many important enzymes, called cupro-enzymes, which speed up the body's energy-yielding (oxidation) reactions. It is also intimately involved in healing processes, excretion of certain toxins (purines), maintaining connective tissue integrity and in the formation of red blood cells. A deficiency of this element can lead to a lowered resistance to infections. Chromium has been observed to be useful in the treatment of pancreatic cancer.

Level of evidence

The importance of minerals to the optimum functioning of bodily systems such as the immune systems has been studied through a great number of pure science and laboratory studies.

Source and price

Neways International has formulated a liquid multi-vitamin and mineral product called Maximol Solution. This liquid contains 67 essential and trace minerals, 17 essential vitamins, 21 amino acids and three enzymes. To provide greater absorption of all of these ingredients into the circulatory system, Maximol has been formulated with organic fulvic acid. Fulvic acid has been identified as playing a key role for the absorption of minerals and nutrients in plants and animals. By providing the minerals in a micro-colloidal state the minerals are much easier to absorb and utilise in the body.

Maximol costs £24.43 for a month's supply. It should be taken at the level of the recommended daily dose.

Most vitamin companies also produce multi-mineral tablets and these, too, should be taken at the recommended daily dose.

Flaxseed oil

Background

Flaxseed oil is also known as linseed oil. It is a very rich source of alpha-linolenic acid (ALA), an important omega-3 fatty acid.

Uses and dosage

Flaxseed oil is used to promote immune system and tissue functioning to improve the body's defences against cancer.

A typical recommended amount of pure virgin, cold-pressed flaxseed oil is 1-2 tablespoons per day. Flaxseed tablets are taken at the levels of 1.5 grams per day.

How to use

It should be bought as cold-pressed (unrefined) flaxseed oil. It has a short shelf life, so must be purchased as fresh as possible and always kept tightly sealed in the fridge. Since flaxseed oil is highly unsaturated, it readily oxidises when exposed to the open air. It should be sold in dark coloured glass bottles as it also breaks down with exposure to light.

It can be self-administered and is taken with food, either as oil in dressings on salads or poured onto hot food after cooking. Never heat flaxseed oil as this will destroy its beneficial properties. It can also be taken in the form of freshly ground linseeds or as capsules/tablets.

Drug interactions and special precautions

None reported.

Mechanism of action

The omega-3 fatty acid in flaxseed/linseed oil, which is called alpha-linolenic acid (ALA), helps maintain the levels of health-promoting eicosanoids (biological activators that regulate all biological activities) and inhibit the production of tumour-promoting eicosanoids. ALA enhances immune function and cellular oxygen use, thereby helping to inhibit tumour growth.

Level of evidence

A $20 million study by the National Cancer Institute (NCI) in 1990 found that flaxseed oil, but not fish oil, reduced the growth of breast cancers and metastases in laboratory animals, when compared to cancerous growth in animals receiving corn oil.[5] Although the NCI study was halted before completion, it determined that flaxseed oil exerts a strong anti-cancer effect, provided the particular oil is high in lignans. Flaxseed oil has been found to contain up to 100 times more lignans than many other plant foods. Animal studies showed that test subjects receiving flaxseed oil experienced a significant reduction in tumour size and number (greater than 50% reduction) after 1-2 months.

Once in the gastrointestinal tract, lignans are converted into enterolactone and enterodiol, which are believed to be the compounds in flaxseed with the anti-cancer effect. Researchers have found that lignans can bind to oestrogen receptors in the body and usefully obstruct the cancer-enhancing effects of oestrogen on breast tissue.

Source and price

Flaxseed oil can be purchased in a bottle and typically costs between £6 and £12 per month. It is available in most good health food stores.

Coenzyme Q10

Background

Coenzyme Q10, also known as ubiquinone, is a benzoquinone compound naturally synthesised by the human body. The Q and 10 in the name refer to the quinone chemical group and the 10 isoprenyl chemical subunits, respectively. Coenzyme Q10 is present in most tissues, as it is an essential component of our energy producing system. The highest concentrations are found in the heart, the liver, the kidneys and the pancreas, where high levels of metabolic activity are maintained continously.[6] Tissue levels of this compound decrease with age and highly stressed lifestyles, due to increased requirements, or insufficient intake of the chemical precursors needed for its synthesis. The ensuing deficiency contributes to ageing and disease processes.

Uses and dosage

For the cancer patient the primary role of Coenzyme Q10 is to help increase energy levels, reduce free-radical damage in the body and increase white cell activity. The dose range is from 90 to 400 mg daily. 90mg per day is taken as a maintenance dose if the condition is stable whereas 400mg per day is taken if there is active cancer in the body.

How to use

Coenzyme Q10 can be self-administered.

Drug interactions and special precautions

Patients undergoing adriamycin chemotherapy should not take Coenzyme Q10 concurrently as it may increase tissue levels of a potentially toxic metabolite of this chemotherapeutic agent. However, if taken before and after adriamycin, it has been shown to reduce the toxicity of adriamycin on heart tissue

Mechanism of action

Coenzyme Q10 is used by the cells of the body in a process called aerobic metabolism. Through this process, energy for cell growth and maintenance is created inside the cells in compartments called mitochondria. Coenzyme Q10 is also used as an antioxidant to protect cells from free-radical damage.

Level of evidence

In patients with cancer, Coenzyme Q10 has been shown to protect the heart from anthracycline-induced cardiotoxicity [7] and to stimulate the immune system.[8] It appears that Coenzyme Q10 has an indirect anti-cancer activity through its effect on the immune system. Stimulation of the immune system by this compound has also been observed in animal studies and in humans without cancer. The ability to protect the heart and enhance the immune system make Coenzyme Q10 a valuable part of alternative treatment particularly if a patient is receiving, or has received, chemotherapy.

Inositol/IP6

Background

This natural substance is a constituent of vitamin B.

Uses and dosage

It is used for the prevention and treatment of cancer. The dose range is from 3 to 6 grams daily in three doses. The higher level is for active treatment of cancer and the lower for maintenance, once remission has been achieved by conventional or holistic methods.

How to use

Inositol can be self-administered and is excellent to revive immune function during and after chemotherapy and also as part of a holistic Health Creation Programme.

Drug interactions and special precautions

None reported.

Mechanism of action

Inositol has a very powerful immune stimulant property, stimulating particularly the production of vital NK killer cells, whilst also raising white cell numbers and activity generally.

It is found in virtually all cells of the body and helps the liver to remove excess fat from its tissues, preventing liver stagnation from fat and bile accumulation.

Level of evidence

John Potter PhD, a researcher at Fred Hutchinson Cancer Research centre in Seattle, Washington, has identified inositol hexaphosphate (IP6) as one of 15 different classes of phytochemicals that have shown anti-cancer activity.[9]

It has also been shown to have direct and indirect immune stimulant properties

Source and price

120 IP6 tablets of 880 mg – £21.95 per month.

414 g of IP6 powder £69.95.

2 Herbal extracts and plant derivatives

Aloe Vera

Background

Aloe Vera is a member of the Lily family and has spiny, fleshy white-speckled leaves. The plant is indigenous to Sudan and the Arabian peninsula but is often grown as a houseplant worldwide.

Uses and dosage

Aloe Vera has long been used medicinally for healing cuts, burns and various skin problems. For the cancer patient, this makes it ideal for preventing skin damage from radiotherapy.

Aloe Vera also soothes and heals internal mucus membranes and is taken as Aloe Vera Juice, one tablespoon three times per day, to help heal the gut lining during and after chemotherapy. It will also help with radiation cystitis at this dosage.

Aloe Vera is also believed to be active in treating cancer directly if taken in large enough doses. For this direct anti-cancer effect take up to 200 ml juice per day in divided doses.

How to use

It is perfectly safe to self-administer Aloe Vera cream, juice or tablets. The use of Aloe Vera during conventional cancer treatment is positively recommended. It can be also used directly from the broken surface of an aloe leaf. Use twice daily on affected skin and continue for up to six weeks after radiotherapy has finished.

Drug interactions and special precautions

None reported.

Mechanism of action

Aloe Vera contains a variety of vitamins, minerals, amino acids, essential fats and enzymes. However, its most potent constituent appears to be acemannan. This water-soluble compound has been found to enhance immune function in mice by increasing the numbers and activity of T-cells and macrophages.[10]

Whilst the therapeutic efficacy of acemannan for human cancer remains to be proven, the compound has demonstrated some interesting anti-cancer activity in animals.[11] The anti-tumour activity seems to be in part due to its ability to inhibit the formation of new cancer cells, the clumping of platelets, and the production of harmful eicosanoids and inflammatory reactions.[12]

Level of evidence

Aloe Vera has a strong anecdotal or folk medicine tradition that is increasingly supported by pure science.

Source and price

Aloe Vera cream is widely available.

Aloe Vera juice – use Aloe Gold from Nature's Own/Cytoplan. This has the highest level of aloe of any proprietary brand (at the time of printing).

High strength Aloe Vera tablets are £3.79 per month from health food shops.

Amygdalin (or Laetrile)

Background

Among alternative cancer physicians Amygdalin is one of the most widely used supplements and there have been numerous positive reports of Amygdalin's therapeutic effectiveness against cancer.

Amygdalin is one of the many nitrilosides, which are cyanide-containing substances found in numerous foods, including the seeds of apricots, apples, cherries, plums and peaches.

Uses and dosage

When the natural substance called Amygdalin is purified and concentrated for use in anti-cancer therapy, it is called Laetrile. For the cancer patient, it is claimed that Laetrile targets only the cancer cells and destroys them through an enzyme process involving cyanide.

Dr Schachter of the Schachter Centre of Complementary Medicine in New York who has used Amygdalin for more than 20 years with cancer patients, indicates that Amygdalin can be taken safely as an oral supplement, at the level of 500 mg, one to three times daily. It may also be administered safely intravenously. By eating Amygdalin-rich foods, patients may get substantial amounts in their diet. One source is bitter apricot kernels that appear safe at the rate of three to five apricot kernels three times per day.

The injectable form is more concentrated enabling the delivery of higher doses in a shorter period of time. After several weeks, if the patient responds well to treatment, the physician will reduce the dosage and prescribe tablets to replace injections. This therapy is usually used in conjunction with the proteolytic enzymes and a diet of fresh fruit and vegetables, whole grains and the elimination of meat and diary products for the duration of the treatment.

How to use

For the initial treatment intravenous, injections need to be administered by a qualified medical practitioner. Subsequent treatment or initial treatment involving an oral dosage of Amygdalin tablets and apricot kernels for nutritional support may be undertaken at home.

Drug interactions and special precautions

It is essential not to take too much Laetrile as cyanide is a poison. Always take Laetrile under medical guidance. Brown, Wood and Smith observed no toxic effects from consistent Amygdalin usage both in mice or humans.[13]

Mechanism of action

Amygdalin consists of two sugar molecules, a benzaldehyde ring and a cyanide radical. The two sugar molecules are split off by the enzyme beta glucosidase (which is found in high levels in cancer cells) and are replaced by glucuronic acid. This results in a selective toxicity to cancer cells and relative non-toxicity to normal cells because the enzyme glucuronidase, which splits off the glucuronic acid, is low in normal cells. The glucuronic acid and the remaining benzaldehyde are then split off from the cyanide molecule, which is then toxic to the cancer cell.

An additional mechanism that protects normal cells from cyanide is that they contain an enzyme known as rhodanase. This enzyme adds a sulphur atom to any free cyanide to form thiocyanate, a relatively harmless substance. Cancer cells do not have significant amounts of this enzyme and are therefore believed to be more susceptible to cyanide poisoning.

Level of evidence

Unfortunately this compound has been subject to much controversy over the years. According to Dr Ralph Moss, research findings on Amygdalin have been consistently suppressed by the pharmaceutical industry, allegedly because the substance is non-patentable.

Amygdalin has been found to have direct anti-cancer potential, particularly with regard to secondary cancers, where a 60% reduction in animal lung metastases has been reported.[14]

Source and price

World Without Cancer, Inc. No 303, 111 Kane Concourse, Bay Harbor Island, Florida, 33154, USA.

International telephone orders: 001 305 861 0898

Internet ordering: www.worldwithoutcancer.com

Prices for treatment in alternative clinics vary and are available upon enquiry. Typically: initial 21 days' intravenous injections is approximately £480, initial 21 days' oral tablets is approximately £300. Subsequent treatment for next three months is approximately £800.

Astragalus

Background

Astragalus is the root of the Astragalus membranaceus plant that is a member of the pea family. It is native to north-east China.

Uses and dosage

Astragalus has long been used as a traditional Chinese medication to treat viral infections. Since 1975 Astragalus has been used in China for cancer patients undergoing radiation treatment and chemotherapy. It appears to help reduce the side-effects, promote immune function and increase survival time.

Astragalus appears particularly useful in cases where the immune system has been damaged by chemicals or radiation, for example, in patients undergoing chemotherapy and/or radiation treatment.

Astralagus is taken orally as a tincture, tablet, capsules or powdered herb. The dose is 3-6 grams per day of the dried root or 250 mg twice daily of the concentrated root extract.

How to use

Astralagus may be self-administered and is safe to use alongside conventional cancer treatment.

Drug interactions and special precautions

None reported.

Mechanism of action

Clinical studies in China have shown Astragalus to be effective when used as a preventive measure against the common cold. Research in animals indicates that Astragalus seems to work by stimulating several aspects of the functioning of the immune system. Phagocytic activity of monocytes and macrophages; interferon production, natural killer cell activity; T cell activity; and other antiviral mechanisms are all increased.[15,16,17]

The active constituents of Astragalus are complex polysaccharides known as saponin glycosides, astraglycosides, flavinoid glycosides and aglycones. These polysaccharides have been found to stimulate the immune system.

Astralagus has also been found to help reverse chemotherapeutically induced immuno-suppression with the drug cyclophosphamide.[18]

Level of evidence

Most of the data relating to clinical efficacy is derived from Chinese studies. There have been several clinical studies providing evidence to support the use of Astragalus for stimulating the immune system.

Source and price

100 capsules (470 mg) approximately £11 per month from health food shops.

Carctol

Background

Carctol is a herbal formulation developed by Dr Nandlal Tiwari based in Jaipur, Rajasthan, India. Each capsule contains the herbs, Hemidesmus Indcus, Tribulus Terrestris, Piper Cubeba Linn, Ammani Vesicatoria, Lepidium Sativum Linn, Blepharis Edulis, Smilax China Linn, Rheum Emodi Wall. Dr Tiwari has been treating cancer with carctol for more than 20 years with some very notable success.

Uses and dosage

Carctol is used by Dr Tiwari as a sole agent. It is taken orally as capsules at the level of 2 capsules 4 times daily (for a 70 kg person) taken after meals and before bed. Whilst taking Carctol, Dr Tiwari advises a vegetarian diet and dietary restrictions that prohibits the consumption of sour and acidic food and drink. Patients must also consume large quantities of boiled refrigerated water (up to 6 pints, 3 litres daily), avoid constipation, and take a digestive enzyme with each dose of the medication.

How to use

Some of the herbs within Carctol are classed as medicines, which means that in the UK it is classed as a medicine and a doctor has to provide a prescription. Because it has not been put through the process of getting a licence as a medicine (which costs millions of pounds) it is therefore an unlicensed medicine. However, a doctor is allowed to prescribe an unlicensed medicine for a patient if he or she believes that it will be of benefit. A list of doctors who prescribe Carctol is to be found in the Resource Directory.

Dr Tiwari recommends that the medicine is taken for a minimum of two months before assessing its value. If there is no improvement of general condition or stabilisation of the cancer within this time he advises the cessation of treatment. Carctol can also be taken to help offset the side-effects of chemotherapy and it is safe and beneficial to take Carctol alongside orthodox treatment.

Drug interactions and special precautions

No drug interactions have been reported. Carctol must not be taken if there is severe constipation or any obstruction to the passage of food through the bowel.

Mechanism of action

None of the herbs within Carctol have a direct anti-cancer effect but jointly they have been seen to produce some unexpected remarkable recoveries. It is believed that its effect is in part due to helping change the pH of the body from more acid to more alkaline. The Carctol formulation has been developed to strengthen the immune system, neutralise toxicity produced by chemo-therapeutic agents, support liver and kidney function, improve digestion and weight gain and calm the nervous system. The precise anti-cancer mechanism of action is not known.

Level of evidence

Dr Tiwari has produced a case study of 1,900 patients who have used Carctol, which is available on the website www.anticancerherb.com. Most patients in the study had been pronounced beyond medical help by their conventional medical team. More than 25% of those studied reported a 75-100% improvement in their condition whilst on Carctol, with a further approximately 30% reporting 50-75% improvement. The best results have been seen with those with gastro-intestinal and haematological cancers. Dr Rosy Daniel has been working with this medicine in the UK since February 2000 and has herself begun to witness some remarkable recoveries. There have also been other reported benefits such as increased energy, recovery of appetite, weight gain and general improvement of well-being.

Source and price

Cankut Herbs in Bristol is currently the sole source of Carctol in the UK. Carctol can be obtained from Cankut Herbs only with a doctor's prescription. Their helpline number is 0117 973 6052. It has been the founder, Mrs Amlani's charitable mission to bring the possible benefits of Carctol to the awareness of those with cancer throughout the world. The price of Carctol is approximately £90 per month plus the cost of the digestive enzymes, which is approximately £10 per month. Digestive enzymes are available from health food shops.

Cat's Claw (Uncaria Tomentosa)

Background

Cat's Claw is a vine that grows high into the canopy roof of the Amazon rain forest, and gets its name from the claw-like thorns that protrude from the woody stems. This plant has been used by many tribes in Peru, for the treatment of inflammatory conditions, intestinal ailments, wounds and cancer.

Uses and dosage

Cat's Claw is taken for its immune system boosting properties in relation to treating cancer. It may be taken as tea, powder or capsules. The dosage is 20 mg per day of the root extract up to 60 mg per day in more serious conditions.

How to use

Cat's Claw may be self-administered.

Drug interactions and special precautions

Cat's Claw must not be taken during chemotherapy as it may cause an aggravation in the drop in the level of red blood cells.

Mechanism of action

Recent studies indicate Cat's Claw contains substances that have immune and digestion enhancing properties.[19] These beneficial constituents of Cat's Claw include several types of antioxidant compounds (polyphones, triterpines and the plant steroids beta-sitosterol, stigmasterol and campesterol). The presence of these compounds is believed to account for the antioxidant and anti-tumour properties of Cat's Claw.

Level of evidence

Pure science to study the constituent elements and their properties.

Source and price

90 capsules approximately £6.50 per month from health food stores.

Echinacea

Background

Echinacea is known as purple coneflower, and is a member of the daisy family native to the United States. American Indians traditionally used the root of this herb on cuts, burns and other injuries to prevent infection and its native name is snake root.

Uses and dosage

Echinacea is used as an immune stimulant, particularly to raise resistance to infections. It is also used to decrease inflammation and allergic reactions. The primary role of Echinacea for the cancer patient is to help provide protection against infection, a common and sometimes fatal complication in advanced-stage cancers or when the immune system is compromised after chemotherapy. It is used for approximately six weeks as a potent immune booster and should be started immediately at the onset of a cold or other infection.

The root extract is taken orally as a tincture in water, tablet or capsule at the level of 225 mg twice daily.

How to use

Echinacea may be self-administered.

Drug interactions and special precautions

No interactions are reported. Long-term use of Echinacea is not recommended. Use for approximately six weeks only as an immune tonic.

Mechanism of action

In recent years Echinacea has been shown to act as a potent immune system booster. Echinacea stimulates the production of white blood cells for protection against bacteria and helps the body produce more interferon for increased protection against viruses.

The main active constituents are polysaccharides, betaine, alkalides and echinolone that appear to be key to the plant's immune boosting ability. These increase macrophage production in the body, which are white cells that help to destroy cancer cells.[20]

Level of evidence

A study on a group of healthy men found that after five days of taking 30 drops of Echinacea extract, three times a day, their white blood cells had doubled their activity (phagocytic power).[21]

There is no doubt this herb has well-known immune-stimulant properties. Certain human studies involving patients with inoperable metastatic oesophageal or colorectal cancer have found Echinacea to increase NK cell activity by 221%. In addition, a phyto-chemical in Echinacea, called arabinogalactan, stimulates the tumour-killing activity of macrophages.

In addition to immune support, Echinacea exerts direct antiviral activity and helps prevent the spread of bacteria by inhibiting a bacterial enzyme called hyaluronidase. This enzyme is secreted by bacteria in order to break through the body's first line of defence, the protective membranes such as the skin or mucous membranes, so that the organism can enter the body.

Source and price

100 capsules (250 mg) £6.00 per month. Available from health food shops.

Essiac (or Renee Caisse herbs)

Background

In the 1920s a Canadian nurse named Renee Cassie discovered a non-toxic herbal tea for treating cancer based on a recipe from the Ojibway, a Native American tribe based in Ontario, Canada. She noticed that her native Indian patients were faring much better than her other patients and put this success down to their use of the tea. She went on to publicise the tea's use widely and it is now available as Essiac (which is Caisse spelt backwards), or as Renee Caisse herbs or Floressence.

Use and dosage

The primary role of Essiac for cancer patient is to help provide protection against infection, facilitate detoxification particularly when undergoing chemotherapy and to boost the body's ability to fight cancer. Essiac is usually taken orally as a herbal medicine at the level of 15 ml in 30 ml of water before breakfast and again at night 2 hours after food.

How to use

Essiac can be self-administered and can be used alongside orthodox cancer treatment. Although it can be purchased in tablet, drop and medicine form, Essiac was originally prepared by Rene Caisse as a herbal drink requiring careful preparation. Once the herbal drink has been prepared from the constituent herbs it can be stored in sterilised bottles and refrigerated. Before use the bottle must be shaken well.

Drug interactions and special precautions

No drug interactions reported. Some doctors advise against taking the herbal formula while pregnant.

Mechanism of action

Essiac is formulated from four herbs – Sheep Sorrel (Rumen Acetosella), Burdock Root (Arctium Lappa), Slippery Elm (Ulmus Fulva) and Indian Rhubarb (Rheum Palmatum). Studies of these components have each demonstrated a significant anti-cancer activity.[22]

Emodin, one of the main constituents in rhubarb, has been shown to inhibit various cancer cell lines [23] and to reduce tumour cell numbers and increase survival time in leukaemic mice.[24] Indian rhubarb has also been shown to exhibit immune-boosting properties and to help cleanse the liver of toxic wastes and improve the supply of oxygen to tissues.

Japanese researchers have identified a potent factor in Burdock that can block cell mutation.[25]

Sheep Sorrel has been shown to possess strong anti-tumour activity and other immune-boosting properties.[26]

Slippery Elm is rich in many vitamins and minerals and helps support the healing of mucous membranes.

Level of evidence

Although Essiac has never undergone randomised clinical trials, Caisse and her associates recorded many impressive case histories and anecdotal success stories. The evidence cited above is pure science relating to the constituent elements of the treatment and their likely actions.

Source and price

Essiac is available as a liquid medicine from Argyll Herbs and many health food shops as liquid, powder and tablets.

Garlic

Background

Garlic has long been recognised to benefit the immune system, improve general health, help ward off colds and treat infections of all sorts.

Uses and dosage

For the cancer patient, garlic can help to strengthen the immune system, facilitate detoxifying the liver and reduce free-radical damage due to its high levels of sulphur-containing amino acids. It may also have a direct anti-cancer effect. The dose is 1 clove or 2 grams of fresh raw garlic daily, which is equivalent to 650 mg of garlic powder or 6 mg of allicin and other active constituents. Fresh raw garlic is very good on buttered toast with tahini or in olive oil as a dressing for pasta and salads.

How to use

Garlic can be self-administered and is beneficial to use alongside orthodox cancer treatment. Cooking garlic will lessen the therapeutic benefits.

Drug interactions and special precautions

Garlic has a mild anti-coagulant effect and may effect the dose requirement of anti-coagulant medications.

Mechanism of action

Garlic contains an abundance of sulphur-containing compounds, especially allylic sulphides. Sulphide compounds enhance the action of cellular enzymes capable of neutralizing carcinogens.

Allicin, one of garlic's main biologically active components, is released when garlic is crushed. It has been shown to decrease breast cancer and prostate cancer cell proliferation in laboratory studies.[27] Research into cancer at universities in Pennsylvannia and Texas in the USA has identified two other compounds active against cancer in crushed garlic, which are diallyl-sulphide and S-allyl cysteine.

In addition to containing substances that appear to inhibit the initiation and promotion phases of oncogenesis; garlic seems to strengthen various aspects of the immune system's response to tumours.[28]

Garlic extract appears able to enhance natural killer cell activity, improve the therapeutic ratio between T helper/suppressor cells, stimulate macrophages to greater activity and enable lymphocytes to become even more cytotoxic (cell-killing) against tumours. Garlic may also block the adhesion of cancer cells to the surface of blood vessels, thereby helping to prevent metastases.[29]

Level of evidence

Pure scientific research now highlights garlic's proven ability to work as a cancer inhibitor and valuable addition to alternative cancer therapy. It has also been shown through epidemiological studies to help to prevent cancer.

Source and price

60 high strength (600 mg) enteric-coated tablets £15.00 per month from health food stores or take as raw garlic in dressings and patés.

Green tea (catechins)

Background

Green and black tea is derived from the same plant, Camellia Sinensis. However, only green tea is rich in the flavonal group of polyphenols known as catechins. The fermentation process used in making black tea destroys the biologically active polyphenols of the fresh leaf. The catechins as a chemical group have significant free-radical scavenging properties and are potent antioxidants.

Uses and dosage

Green tea and catechin tablets are used for the prevention and treatment of cancer. When brewing the tea, hot but not boiling water is poured over the leaves. The brewing time is just a minute or two. Boiling water is too harsh for green tea, damaging the flavour and the vital ingredients. It is taken without the addition of milk and sugar.

The tea can be drunk throughout the day in place of ordinary tea as a preventive or treatment of cancer: 4-7 cups per day are recommended. Alternatively, catechins can be taken in tablet form called Te-green made by Pharmanex at the level of 2 tablets of 250 mg, 3 times per day. For prevention, one capsule of Te-green per day is recommended.

How to use

Green tea and catechin tablets can be self-administered. Green tea should be kept in a cool, dry location, avoiding heat and light.

Drug interactions and special precautions

There are some reports of allergic reactions to green tea. Use of catechins during lactation is not advised. It is also mildly anti-coagulant so extra care should be taken by those on anti-coagulant drugs. It is high in potassium and should be avoided by those on a low potassium diet.

Mechanism of action

Green tea contains a substance called epigallocatechin gallate, which has been shown to inhibit the growth of cancers and lowers cholesterol.[30] This is one of a number of chemical compounds known as polyphenolic catechins, which are many times stronger than vitamin E in defending the body against cancer-producing free radicals.[31]

The catechins found in green tea support the immune system's responsiveness and have demonstrated powerful anti-carcinogenic effects.[32] Studies have indicated that green tea can reduce the risk of cancers of the liver and throat.[33] Green tea flavonols (the active bioflavonoids in the tea) and catechin tablets may offer substantial protection if consumed on a regular basis.

Level of evidence

The evidence described above is mainly pure science to establish the constituents and their mechanism of action. There are also epidemiological studies to establish the cancer-preventive properties of green tea.

Source and price

£3-10 per month for tea bags. Green tea can be found in most good health food stores and even in some supermarkets.

The amount of polyphenol activity in green tea leaves varies with respect to climate, season, horticultural practices and the position of the leaf on the harvested shoot. Using a specific process, a green tea concentrate can be prepared by lightly steaming and drying the leaves of the tea plant. This steaming process preserves polyphenol activity. Green tea concentrates are now available as a food supplement in capsule form. The American Pharmanex Corporation manufacturers a green tea concentrate called Te-green, which contains high levels of the polyphenols.

Indole-3-Carbinol

Background

Indole-3-Carbinol (I-3-C) is a compound occurring naturally in cruciferous vegetables such as broccoli, cabbage and brussel sprouts. Consumption of cruciferous vegetables has long been associated with a reduced risk of breast, colon and prostate cancer.

Use and dosage

Indole-3-Carbinol is being proposed as a possible natural alternative to Tamoxifen, the oestrogen-blocking drug, which is taken by many breast cancer patients to prevent stimulation of the growth of their cancer by oestrogen. Indole-3-Carbinol is also recommended for its direct anti-cancer effect and for cancer prevention. It is taken orally as tablets. The effective dose established in human studies is 6-7 mg per kg per day. This amounts to an average dose of around 500 mg per day.

How to use

Indole-3-Carbinol can be self-administered. It can be used safely alongside orthodox cancer treatment.

Drug interactions and special precautions

There are none reported.

Mechanism of action

Indole-3-Carbinol has been shown to boost the production of enzymes that reduce the formation of malignant tissue, promote hormone balance, work with antioxidants to prevent free-radical damage, and detoxify body tissues.

In 1991, researchers at the Institute for Hormone Research in New York found that by using Indole-3-Carbinol they had been able to convert the stronger form of oestrogen (known as oestradiol) into a weaker form (2-hydroxy-estrone) by up to 50%. In women 2-hydroxy-estrone is considered to be a more protective form of oestrogen in the body, as it effectively blocks the strong signals for growth that oestradiol sends to cancer cells.[34]

Researchers at the Strang Cancer Research Laboratory in New York in 1997, found that when Indole-3-Carbinol changes oestradiol into the weaker form of oestrogen, it stops breast cancer cells from growing by up to 60% and provokes the cancer cells to self-destruct.[35]

Subsequent studies at the University of California in Berkeley have shown that Indole-3-Carbinol inhibits a certain type of human breast cancer cell from growing by as much as 90% in laboratory experiments.[36]

Professor Gary Firestone, co-author of a report in the February 13th 1998 issue of the Journal of Biological Chemistry, indicates that Indole-3-Carbinol appears to interfere with the cell cycle by turning off a gene for an enzyme important in the cell's growth cycle, and in so doing, stops the growth of cancer cells without killing normal cells.

Level of evidence

The evidence cited above is pure science relating to the study of the effects of Indole-3-Carbinol in the laboratory. However, the mechanism appears to be a strong one and the potential use of this treatment, especially for women with breast cancer, is compelling.

Source and price

60 capsules (250 mg) £39.95 per month.

Iscador (Mistletoe)

Background

Iscador is the trade name for a mistletoe preparation that has been used by European physicians since 1920 for the treatment of cancer. Iscador consists of fermented extracts of European mistletoe and was originally developed by an Austrian scientist called Rudolf Steiner, who pioneered the speciality known as Anthroposophical Medicine. There are several different types of Iscador dependent on which type of tree the mistletoe grows on.

Uses and dosage

Iscador is used by people with cancer to stimulate the immune system and inhibit tumour formation. Iscador is usually injected. The dose is individually determined.

How to use

Iscador has to be prescribed by a doctor and it is best to see an anthroposophical or homeopathic doctor for this purpose. Once prescribed at the right level and type for a given individual, the Iscador can be used at home. This means either learning to inject yourself, much like a diabetic does, or getting your local practice nurse or GP to do it. Occasionally it is prescribed in drop form, most commonly when there is a brain tumour or brain secondaries. There is often an initial flu-like illness when treatment begins, which is evidence that a strong immune reaction is being provoked in the body. Usually, Iscador is not used at the same time as orthodox cancer medicine.

Drug interactions and special precautions

Iscador is safe for use when given at the right dose but can cause adverse reactions if taken in excess. It is therefore important to use under the supervision of a properly trained anthroposophical or homeopathic doctor.

Mechanism of action

The therapeutic success of Iscador has been reported in nearly 5,000 cases studied. In animal experiments, Iscador has been found to kill cancer cells, stimulate the immune system and significantly inhibit tumour formation.[37]

The activity of various immune cells increases significantly within 24 hours of injecting Iscador.[38] These effects are likely to explain the findings that Iscador selectively inhibits the growth of different types of tumour cells.[39]

Level of evidence

The evidence for the effectiveness of Iscador is of a high quality. Randomised controlled clinical trials have been judged to be clinically significant. There is also very compelling laboratory evidence as well as strong anecdotal evidence for the use of Iscador.

Source and price

Iscador can be obtained on NHS prescription if prescribed by a GP, consultant or specialist anthroposophical or homeopathic doctor. The main distributor of Iscador in this country is Weleda, Heanor Road, Ilkeston, Derbyshire, telephone 0115 944 8200 who are the major anthroposophical suppliers in the UK. They do an 'Iscador Patient Pack', which contains all the relevant information about getting on to Iscador plus a countrywide list of anthroposophical doctors. Most of these doctors will prescribe Iscador on an outpatient basis. Iscador is also prescribed by doctors at the Homeopathic Hospitals in London, Bristol and Glasgow.

The main anthroposophical clinic in the UK is Park Attwood in Worcestershire, where you can go to be put on to Iscador over a two-week in-patient stay with doctor and nurse supervision, telephone 01299 861444. This costs £204 per day, which includes doctor appointments and sessions of massage, movement and art therapy as well as nurse treatments with herbal compresses and aromatherpy. On leaving you will be given a month's supply of Iscador. Park Attwood is keen that no-one is denied access to their services on financial grounds and will help those who cannot afford the fees to try to obtain help to meet the costs.

Iscador injections bought privately cost approximately £6 each and about three are required per week whilst on treatment. If obtained with an NHS prescription they can be obtained for the prescription charge alone.

Mushrooms and their extracts

Background

Many mushrooms we know to have anti-cancer properties. The most commonly used mushrooms in alternative cancer treatments are Maitake, Shiitake, Coriolus Versicolor and Reishi.

Uses and dosage

The primary role of these mushrooms for the cancer patient is their immune-boosting properties. These mushrooms are available as powders, with the therapeutic dose being about 500 mg three times a day. Maitake mushroom extract is also available as MGM3 and the dose range is 3-6 grams per day in three divided doses. The 6 gram level is for those who have been recently diagnosed or who have cancer present within the body, and the 3 gram level is for those whose condition is stable. The dose of Coriolus is usually 1 capsule three times per day before food, but can go right up to 9 capsules 3 times per day in those who are very immuno-compromised.

How to use

The mushrooms are eaten fresh or taken medicinally as a liquid extract or powder. Mushrooms are self-administered and can be used alongside conventional cancer treatment.

Drug interactions and special precautions

There are occasionally allergic reactions to these mushrooms but no reported drug interactions.

Mechanism of action

The Maitake mushroom has been shown to exhibit potent activity against cancer, inhibiting both carcinogenesis and metastasis, according to Hiroaki Nanba, PhD, of the Department of Immunology at Kobe Womens's College of Pharmacy in Kobe, Japan. Animal research suggests the Maitake supplements increase the body's ability to destroy tumours.[40]

Research has shown the Shiitake mushroom contains an anti-tumour polysaccharide called lentinan, which appears to activate T lymphocytes, macrophages and other immune cells that mediate the release of cytokines. Lentinan has also shown potential anti-tumour activity in humans when given both orally and by injection. It is presently being studied as an adjuvant treatment to protect cells from the cytotoxic effects of chemotherapy agents.[41]

Compounds in each of these mushrooms increase the tumour-fighting activity of NK cells and improve antibody responses, but maitake seems to have the strongest and most consistent effect.

Coriolus is the mushroom most favoured by alternative cancer doctor Julian Kenyon and is available from his Dove Clinic. He believes it is the strongest immune stimulant mushroom. Reishi has been extremely investigated by Pharmanex and their product Reishi-max is available from their UK distributors, Nu-Skin.

Level of evidence

The evidence described above is pure science and case study as the effects of these mushrooms have been studied both in the laboratory and in humans.

Source and price

The mushrooms can sometimes be bought from oriental food suppliers, or even good greengrocers. Maitake and Shiitake mushroom extracts are available fresh or dried, in capsules or tinctures and are available in specialist health food stores. The liquid extract is available from the Nutri Centre where 30 ml costs £39.95. 120 capsules of the powdered extract costs £29.95. Coriolus is available from the Dove Clinic. The cost of MGM3 is £64.95 for 50 capsules of 250 mg.

Noni juice

Background

The Noni plant (Morinda Citrifolia) is a tropical plant indigenous to areas of Australia, Malaysia and Polynesia. The plant has a long history of medicinal use throughout these areas. It has traditionally been used by people in the South Pacific as a remedy to treat a variety of ailments. The plant is a small, blossoming shrub with rounded branches and dark green glossy leaves that measure approximately a foot in length. Clusters of small white flowers sprout at different times and eventually evolve into bumpy egg-shaped fruit that are a few inches long. Noni juice is made from this fruit.

Use and dosage

The primary role of Noni juice for the cancer patient is to help strengthen the immune system to combat cancer and provide protection against infection. Noni may be taken as fruit juice, tea or as tablets. The dosage depends on the condition of the patient.

How to use

Noni juice is self-administered and can be used alongside conventional treatment. Ideally Noni extracts should be taken on an empty stomach approximately half an hour before meals twice daily. The process of digesting food is believed to interfere with the medicinal value of the alkaloid compounds contained in the juice.

Drug interactions and special precautions

There are no reported drug interactions. If the dose is too high then the side-effects of burping and loose stools can occur. This can be prevented by lowering the dose.

Mechanism of action

Over 140 active constituents have been identified in different parts of the Noni plant. The juice contains a wide variety of substances including vitamin C, selenium, sodium, potassium, polysaccharides and many useful phyto-chemicals.

Scientific studies investigating Noni as an anti-cancer agent have been encouraging.[42,43] A study conducted in 1994, highlighted the anti-cancer activity of Noni against lung cancer in mice. A team of scientists from the university of Hawaii used live laboratory mice to test the medicinal properties of the Noni fruit against Lewis Lung Carcinomas that were artificially transferred to their lung tissue.[44] The mice left untreated died in 9 to 12 days. However, those mice that were given Noni juice in consistent daily dosages lived significantly longer. Almost half of these lived for more than 50 days. This study was duplicated several times with equivalent results. The average survival time was 123% longer in the Noni group. The scientists discovered that the Noni juice contained a polysaccharide compound called 6-D-glucopyranose penta-acetate. It is this polysaccharide compound that stimulates the activity of macrophages and T-lymphocytes enabling the body's own immune system to attack cancerous cells.

Scientific research on the medicinal uses of Noni was presented at the 83rd, 84th and 85th Annual Meetings of the American Association for Cancer Research. The conference conclusion stated that the chemical constituents of the juice acted indirectly by enhancing the ability of the immune system to deal with the invading malignancy, by boosting macrophage or lymphocyte activity.

Damnacanthal, an anthraquinone compound contained in the fruit has also been shown to block or inhibit the activation of ras oncogenes, which, when activated, can initiate many types of cancers.

Level of evidence

The evidence cited above is based on animal and laboratory studies together with some anecdotal evidence.

Source and price

One litre Hawaiian Noni Juice, £24.68 per month from Healthy Solutions.

Pau D'Arco

Background

Pau D'Arco is a herbal extract from the inner bark of the Tabebuia genus, found in South American rainforests.

Use and dosage

Pau D'Arco is used to treat and prevent cancer. It is taken orally as capsules or powdered dry bark. The dosage may vary according to the condition of the patient, but patients usually take 250 mg tablet three times per day with meals.

How to use

Pau D'Arco is self-administered and is safe to use alongside conventional cancer treatment.

Drug interactions and special precautions

There are none reported.

Mechanism of action

The main active ingredient is a substance called lapachol – whose molecular composition makes it uniquely suited to induce strong biological activity against cancer.[45]

Level of evidence

In one study nine patients with various cancers (liver, kidney, breast and prostate) were given pure lapachol in 250 mg capsules with meals. All nine patients showed a shrinkage of tumours and reduction in tumour-related pain; three patients experienced complete remissions, and there were no side effects.[46] In studies of mice injected with leukaemia cells, the life-span of animals given lapachol was 80% greater than that of the control group.[47]

Source and price

Pau D'Arco is available from the Nutri Centre at £8.95 for 60 capsules of 100 mg. It is also available in tincture form at a cost of £6.99 for 30 ml.

PC Spes

Background

PC Spes is a combination of 8 medical herbs: Scutellaria Biaicalensis, Glycyrrhiza Glabra, Ganoderma Lucidium, Isatis Indigotica, Panax Pseudo-Ginseng, Serenoa Repens, Dendrantherma Morifolium and Rabdosia Rubescens. All of these are Chinese herbs except Serenoa Repens, which is an extract of the American Dwarf Palm or Saw Palmetto. At the time of writing it is difficult to obtain PC Spes due to recent controversy following the discovery of contaminants in commercially available PC Spes.

Use and dosage

PC Spes has been used extensively by men with prostate cancer to arrest the progression of the disease. It may also help treat lymphoma, leukaemia, breast cancer and melanoma. The active treatment dose is 12 tablets daily, reducing to 6 tablets daily once the PSA marker level has dropped and plateaued in prostate cancer.

How to use

PC Spes can be self-administered. It is taken as tablets and the dose is 12 tablets daily, initially taken as 4 tablets three times per day. This should bring the PSA level down to a new lower level at which it should plateau. Once a new, lower, stable level has been reached, the dose can then be halved to 6 tablets per day, ie two tablets three times per day.

Drug interactions and special precautions

PC Spes has been reported to have 'an acceptable toxicity profile'. It does raise the risk of venous thrombosis by 8% meaning that individuals who are at high clotting risk due to existing vascular disease must be careful with their use of this treatment. It is also inadvisable to take it alongside stilboestrol treatment for prostate cancer, as this itself can carry up to a 35% clotting risk.

Mechanism of action

The combined mixture of herbs contains flavinoids that have antioxidant activity, anti-inflammatory and anti-carcinogenic actions. PC Spes also contains compounds that may enhance immune cell action. It also has components that interfere with testosterone metabolism and prevent testosterone from binding to prostate cells. Acting together in the PC Spes mixture, individual components may team up to block prostate cancer progression, in part by blocking androgen-supported prostate cell growth and by causing cell death.

A recent phase 2 study assessed the efficacy and toxicity of PC Specs in patients with advanced prostate cancer. The study concluded that PC Specs appears to be active against prostate cancer.[48]

Level of evidence

Both pure science, anecdotal and randomised control trials evidence for the use of PC Spes is compelling.

Source and price

The supply of PC Spes has been interrupted at the time of writing due to controversy following the discovery of some medicinal contaminants in PC Spes that has been commercially available. These contaminants have included a warfarin-like compound used to prevent blood clotting and a compound like stilboestrol, which is used in the mainstream treatment of prostate cancer. Efforts are currently being made to re-establish a reliable supply of PC Spes. When available 60 capsules are usually £89.95 from the Nutri Centre. These were formally available more cheaply from the American supplier, Botanics, on 001 516 432 1758.

Turmeric

Background

Turmeric is a member of the ginger family and is native to India and China. It is a major herb in Indian cooking and appears to exert powerful antioxidant effects, sufficient to reduce carcinogenesis.

Use and dosage

The active constituent is called curcumin and it protects against free-radical damage as it is a very strong antioxidant. The primary role of curcumin for the cancer patient is to reduce the amount of free radicals in the body, which can be generated by chemotherapy and radiotherapy.

Curcumin is taken orally as a powder or in capsule form. 400 mg of turmeric is taken three times a day in capsules or tablets.

How to use

Curcumin can be self-administered and can be taken alongside conventional cancer treatment.

Drug interactions and special precautions

Turmeric is safe. It has been used in food for many centuries with no adverse reactions. However, people with gallstones and those who are pregnant should avoid turmeric due to its mild stimulant effect on smooth muscle.

Mechanism of action

The main active component of turmeric is a yellow pigment called curcumin, which possesses both anti-inflammatory and antioxidant properties. Research indicates that turmeric can inhibit cancer at various stages of cancer development.[49] Part of the therapeutic effect may be that curcumin helps reduce the production of PGE2 and other 'bad' eicosanoids that promote tumour growth.[50] Curcumin also plays a role in the production of the carcinogen-detoxifying enzyme, glutathione-S-transferase.

Level of evidence

Research indicates that turmeric can inhibit cancer at various stages of cancer development. After 1 month, smokers who took two tablets containing 750 mg of turmeric daily had a significant reduction in the level of urinary mutagens (from cigarette smoking) whereas the control group's urinary mutagen level remained unchanged.[51] Dietary administration of curcumin suppresses colon tumour size significantly (by more than 57%) and may also inhibit the progression of the cancer.[52]

Source and price

100 capsules (400 mg) £6.50 per month from health food shops.

3 Anti-cancer substances

In addition to the nutrients, herbal and plant extracts, there are a variety of anti-cancer substances being used by forward-looking cancer doctors to treat cancer.

Natural progesterone

Background

Human progesterone is made by the ovaries, adrenal glands and fat cells. Ovarian production stops after menopause. Synthetic progesterone is sometimes used for treating menopausal symptoms and cancer. The Mexican Yam is rich in a natural precursor of progesterone that is turned into progesterone when absorbed into the body, and this substance has come to be known as natural progesterone. The use of this natural progesterone source has been championed by Dr John Lee, who has written several books on the subject. Natural progesterone cream is also used to help prevent hot flushes induced by Tamoxifen as long as the tumour is progesterone negative.

Uses and dosage

Natural progesterone is being used by some women with breast cancer as an alternative to Tamoxifen, the oestrogen-blocking drug if they have an oestrogen positive (progesterone negative) tumour. This puts the body into a state of 'progesterone dominance'. In this state, it is much harder for tissues and tumours that thrive in an 'oestrogen dominant' state to grow.

This fact is evidenced by the discovery that women with breast cancer who are operated on in the second half of their cycle have lower recurrence rates of their cancer and better overall survival rates. This means that when progesterone levels are naturally high in the blood, metastases are less likely to form.

How to use

Natural progesterone is taken either orally or used as a skin cream, which is rubbed into the fine skinned areas of the body, such as the inner arm and inner thigh, at an individually prescribed level. Any patient receiving hormonal therapy should be under medical supervision. Natural progesterone has to be prescribed by a doctor. It is safe to use whilst undergoing conventional cancer treatment.

Drug interactions and special precautions

Progesterone is safe to take with other drugs. Some women do have unacceptable side-effects while on progesterone and the dosage has to be tailored carefully to the individual.

Mechanism of action

Studies have shown that low natural progesterone levels in the body can increase the risk of developing breast cancer. A study was done at the Private Obstetrics and Gynaecology Clinic at the John Hopkins Medical School published in the American Journal of Epidemiology in 1981 to test the hypotheses that progesterone deficiency plays a major role in breast cancer. The study took 20 years to complete following two groups of women: one with normal progesterone levels and one with low progesterone levels.

When the low progesterone group was compared with the normal progesterone group, it was found that the occurrence of breast cancer was 5.4 times greater in the women in the low progesterone group.

In a 1995 study published in the Journal of Fertility and Sterility,[53] researchers did a double-blind randomised study examining the use of topical progesterone (cream) and/or topical oestrogen in relation to breast duct cell growth. Forty premenopausal women scheduled to have breast surgery for removal of a presumably benign lump were studied. They were divided into four groups and asked to apply a gel to their breasts daily for 10 to 13 days before surgery. One group received a placebo, one group received progesterone, one group received oestrogen (estradiol) and one group received a combination of progesterone and oestrogen. Blood tests were taken the day of surgery and breast tissue taken during surgery was tested for hormone levels and the rate of cell growth. The women using progesterone had dramatically reduced cell multiplication rates compared with any of the other groups. The women using a combination of progesterone and oestrogen were closer to the placebo group.

This study provided some of the first direct evidence that both oestradiol and progesterone are well absorbed through the skin, that 10-13 days of transdermal (on the skin) hormone application significantly increases the concentration of hormone levels in breast cells, that estradiol significantly increases breast cell hyperplasia (increased cell growth) and that progesterone decreases cell proliferation rates, even when oestrogen is also supplemented.

Proponents of the benefits of natural progesterone believe that the very high levels of breast cancer in the west are due to women being in a state of oestrogen dominance, due to excess body weight, high animal fat diet and lack of exercise, and they prescribe progesterone to help overcome this risky condition of oestrogen dominance.

Level of evidence

The evidence cited above is high-quality randomised control trial evidence and these arguments for the benefits of natural progesterone must be taken seriously.

Source and price

Progesterone cream is available by doctor's prescription from Higher Nature (telephone 01435 883484) at a cost of £19 per tube for the 1.5% strength and £24 per tube for the 3% strength, and from Healthy Solutions at a cost of £18.82 for 60 ml jar. Progesterone is also available from conventional doctors but this tends to be the synthetic variety, which is reported to have more side-effects such as water retention, weight gain and mood disturbance, which are rarely reported with the natural progesterone cream.

Shark and bovine cartilage

Background

Cartilage is a tough, elastic connective tissue that does not develop a blood supply because it contains various 'anti-angiogenic' substances that prevent the proliferation of blood vessels.

Use and dosage

The main use of shark and bovine cartilage for the cancer patient is their ability to inhibit the development of new blood vessels in a developing tumour.

Cartilage is taken orally as capsules or powder. Sometimes it is taken as the oil extract. To get more pronounced effects Dr Lane, the main pioneer of the use of shark's cartilage, recommends the use of 1 gram of the powder per kg body weight per day. Bovine cartilage is usually given at lower levels than this.

How to use

Cartilage can be self-administered but it is very unpalatable due to its taste. Ideally it should be used under medical supervision.

Drug interactions and special precautions

No drug interactions have been reported.

Please note: IT IS VITAL NOT TO TAKE SHARK'S CARTILAGE WHEN PREGNANT AS IT CAN INHIBIT THE PROPER DEVELOPMENT OF THE BLOOD SUPPLY TO THE BABY IN THE PLACENTA.

Mechanism of action

To grow, all tumours require the development of new blood vessels, a process known as angiogenesis. Significant interest in shark cartilage was generated in 1992 by the release of the book called 'Sharks Don't Get Cancer' by Dr William Lane. He highlighted that shark cartilage does not contain any blood vessels and its protein component has strong angiogenesis-inhibiting properties. Before this, there was already compelling literature about the possible role of bovine cartilage as an angiogenesis-inhibiting factor. This can prevent new blood vessel formation as a tumour grows, thereby cutting off its supply of nutrients and therefore its ability to grow. The cartilage approach, when combined with other immune-enhancing agents, has proved a useful addition in helping to reduce tumour growth and induce remission. In mainstream medicine, trials are underway with the angiogenesis-inhibiting drug Thalidomide.

Level of evidence

Dr Lane reports that shark cartilage appears effective against solid tumours and has seen tumour reduction rates of 15–67% in advanced prostate tumours.

In 1990, a Japanese researcher, T. Oikawa further confirmed the clinical benefits of shark cartilage by finding a 'significant inhibition of angiogenesis' with the substance.[54] Shark's cartilage is currently being tested by the American FDA for clinical efficacy.

Source and price

45 capsules £15.09 per month. 250 grams of powder £44.25 from the Nutri Centre.

Hydrazine sulphate

Background

Hydrazine sulphate is a synthetic chemical developed by Dr Joseph Gold based in Syracuse, New York. Its use has been controversial – especially in the USA.

Uses and dosage

Hydrazine sulphate appears to inhibit the severe weight loss, which is associated with serious cancer. It is also believed to have indirect anti-tumour effects. Dosage is typically 60 mg capsules, 3 to 4 times per day after meals.

How to use

Hydrazine sulphate can be self-administered and is taken orally as tablets. However, medical supervision is recommended.

Drug interactions and special precautions

Please note: HYDRAZINE SULPHATE MUST NOT BE USED IN CONJUNCTION WITH ALCOHOL, ANTI-DEPRESSANTS, SLEEPING PILLS OR TRANQUILLISERS.

Pain medications may be safely used without interaction with Hydrazine sulphate, but dosages of more than 25 mg of vitamin B6 and more than 3 grams of vitamin C per day may interfere with Hydrazine sulphate's activity.

Mechanism of action

Dr Gold points out that the weight loss caused by the cancer process can often be more life threatening than the invasiveness of the tumour itself. The weight loss seen in cancer is called cachexia, which means weight loss due to loss of lean tissue and muscle mass as well as fat. Advanced cancer tumours appear to grow at the expense of the body's healthy tissue. The constant high metabolic demand of the growing tumours uses up first the body's fat and sugar reserves and then the muscle and protein reserves.

By blocking a particular enzyme in the liver that is involved in the generation of glucose from other substances, Hydrazine sulphate can inhibit this weight loss process. Hydrazine sulphate also improves the appetite, increases the sense of well-being, and often results in weight gain in those who have lost weight. It may also contribute directly to the shrinkage of the tumour by helping to deprive it of its glucose supply.

Level of evidence

Research on Hydrazine sulphate indicates it leads to significant subjective improvements (notably in controlling pain and nausea) as well as to favourable clinical outcomes for many types of cancer.[55]

A study of 740 cancer patients (200 with lung cancer, 138 with stomach cancer, 66 with breast cancer, 31 with melanoma and other) reported tumour stabilisation or regression in 51% of patients, while 46.6% of the patients reported symptomatic improvements such as fewer respiratory problems and a decrease in fever.[56]

For more clinical information about Hydrazine sulphate contact Syracuse Research Institute, Joseph Gold, MD, 600 East Genesee Street, Syracuse, New York 13202 USA. Telephone 001 315 472 6616.

Source and price

100 capsules (60 mg) £52.50 per month available from the Nutri Centre.

Urea

Background

Urea is produced naturally by the liver as a waste product of protein metabolism. The use of urea in cancer treatments was pioneered by Professor E V Danopoulas, of the Medical School of Athens University.

Use and dosage

Urea has been used for treating liver cancer and preventing the development of metastases or secondary tumours in the liver as this is the only organ that shows high concentrations of urea after oral ingestion. This therapy may not be effective against cancers other than those of the liver. The dose is individually determined.

How to use

Urea can be taken orally, as tablet or powder, which can be self-administered. Urea is also injected, which requires medical administration. It is recommended that urea therapy is taken under medical supervision.

Drug interactions and special precautions

None reported.

Mechanism of action

The theory behind urea therapy is that it alters the chemical properties of the cellular surfaces around malignant tumour cells, thereby disrupting the processes necessary for uncontrolled cellular growth.[57]

Level of evidence

Professor E F Demopoulas at the Medical school of Athens University has used this substance to treat cancer patients. Dr Demopoulas found that injections of a 50% urea solution directly into a mass of large, fast growing tumours was effective, and injections around the tumour site were even more effective.[58] Significant healing responses were reported in 15 of 22 patients diagnosed with cancer that had metastasised to the liver.[59] This is case study rather than randomised controlled trial evidence.

Source and price

Urea is available in a powder form (in a formula with creatine monohydrate) from: Innovative Therapeutics, 2020 Franklin Street, Carlyle, IL 62231, USA. Telephone 001 888 688 9922.

4 Adrenaline therapy

Background

German alternative cancer medicine pioneer, Waldraut Fryda, believes that cancer arises in the body due to adrenal exhaustion. This then causes a chain reaction, causing the thyroid to attempt to compensate, ultimately becoming 'burned out'. The knock-on effects on the immune and endocrine systems then leave the door open for cancer development. The treatment involves correcting the disruption in neuro-endocrine function and stimulating adrenal gland regeneration.

Use and dosage

Adrenaline therapy is initially set up by a doctor and thereafter involves self-administration of injections and supplements.

Drug interactions and special precautions

None known.

Mechanism of action

A detailed explanation of Dr Fryda's theory is available in her book, 'Adrenaline deficiency as the cause of cancer' pub. Kunst & Altag (4th ed).

Level of evidence

The authors are not aware of any scientific evidence for this approach at present. However, there is anecdotal evidence for the use of this therapy.

Source and price

In the UK, adrenaline therapy is performed by Dr Fritz Schellander and Dr Julian Kenyon. Dr Fryda is virtually retired, but does conduct the therapy personally with small numbers of clients, by referral from the UK's holistic and alternative cancer doctors.

5 Vaccine therapies

The body's immune system plays a critical role in the combating of cancer. Specific vaccine immunotherapy techniques designed to support, enhance or restore optimal immune function can potentially help the body's ability to stabilise and reverse the cancer without the adverse side-effects associated with conventional therapies. The following vaccine therapies are all designed to stimulate the immune system to combat cancer – either non-specifically with vaccines such as Coley's toxins or the BCG vaccine, or specifically with vaccines that are made from cancer tissue directly.

Coley's toxins

Background

In the 1920s, Dr William Coley proposed that the rise in immune activity caused by certain infectious bacterial diseases, might stimulate a useful immune response against malignancies. He introduced the bacterial challenge into the body in the form of a sterilized vaccine. Dr Coley found his 'toxins' could give the bodies defences a non-specific 'kick start' against cancer cells which would produce more white cells to attack the cancer as well as the bacteria.

Source and price

For more information about Coley's toxins contact Innovative Therapeutics, 2020 Franklin Street, Carlyle, IL 62231, USA. Telephone 001 888 688 9922.

BCG

More currently the BCG vaccine is used to stimulate a non-specific rise in immune function on the same principles as the Coley's toxins.

Melanoma vaccine

A great deal of work has been done on vaccines for people with melanoma. This was pioneered at the John Wayne Clinic in California and has been the specialist area of interest of Professor Gus Dalgleish of St George's Hospital, London. Melanoma vaccines are made either from the person with melanoma's own tumour tissue or from melanoma tissue previously collected from another person with the disease. Professor Dalgleish has since extended his use of vaccines to many other types of cancer, and is pioneering dendritic cell therapy in the UK, as is alternative medicine doctor Julian Kenyon at the Dove Clinic.

Dendritic cell therapy

New excitement is being generated in the field of cancer medicine, mainstream and alternative, through the advent of dendritic cell therapy for people with cancer. This involves priming of the individual's dendritic cells with tumour antigen in order to reactivate the body's own immune reaction to the tumour. This helps because in most people with cancer, their immune system has become unable to recognise, and therefore fight, cancer cells. Dendritic cell therapy will greatly amplify the effect of all other therapies aimed at immune stimulation as it will make the re-activated immune system much more tumour specific. Professor Dalgleish is available to help with appropriate private medical referrals.

Source and price

Dendritic cell therapy is available in the UK from Dr Julian Kenyon at the Dove Clinic for Integrated Medicine in Winchester and Harley Street, London. The cost is available on enquiry. Dr Kenyon collects tumour antigen from urine after treating the individual with high dose vitamin C treatment given intravenously. Dendritic cell therapy is also available from Dr Thomas Nesselhut in Germany who collects the necessary antigen and cells from blood samples – a technique favoured by some immunologists (telephone 0049 552 72056). Again, the cost is available on enquiry. Professor Dalgleish is available to help with appropriate private medical referral.

Immuno-augmentative therapy

Immuno-augmentative therapy (IAT) was developed in the 1960s by Dr Lawrence Burton, a cancer researcher at the California Institute of Technology. Dr Burton isolated four blood protein components in mice that were capable of crossing the species barrier and producing cancer remissions is humans. According to Dr Burton's theory, when the four blood protein components are balanced, the body should be able to subdue cancer cells; but if any of the components are out of balance, the body cannot adequately defend itself. The aim of his therapy is therefore to give the correct balance of these factors to humans to combat cancer.

According to Dr Burton's records, IAT has shown good results as a treatment for cancers of the bladder, prostate, pancreas and lymphomas.[60]

Source

Although Dr Burton died in 1993, IAT is still offered today at the clinic he founded in Freeport on Grand Bahama Island. For more information on IAT contact IAT Centre in Grand Bahama on 001 242 352 4755.

TVZ-7 lymphocyte treatment

While Coley's toxins and Burton's immuno-augmentative therapy are examples of non-specific imunotherapy, TVZ-7 is an example of specific immunotherapy. In TVZ-7, particular components of the immune system are targeted and activated for a more precise response. Dr Ravi Devgan of Toronto, Canada, has used TVZ-7 with his patients and has seen positive results. He indicates it is one of the most potent immune modulators he is aware of.

Source

For more information on TVZ-7 contact Integrated Biologics in the USA on 001 860 963 2612.

T/Tn antigen breast cancer vaccine

Cancer cells have proteins, or antigens, on their surfaces that can be recognised by the immune system. The identification of certain cancer-related antigens forms the basis of this approach developed by Dr Georg Springer. Dr Springer showed that two antigens, called T and Tn play a vital role in the immune system's ability to respond to cancer. Since the early 1980s, Dr Springer has repeatedly shown that the immune system's reaction to T and Tn antigens results in strong cancer cell-killing activity in both animal and human studies.[61]

Using various biochemical tests. Dr Springer has detected the T and Tn antigens in more than 90% of all cancers. The less aggressive cancers (meaning they are well differentiated) produce a higher proportion of the T antigen, while the Tn antigen predominates in the more aggressive cancers (meaning they are poorly differentiated).[62]

Through the use of a specially developed vaccine, Dr Springer demonstrated that the immune system's reaction to T and Tn antigens results in much enhanced cancer-cell killing activity.

Direct cancer vaccines are also being pioneered by Professor Gus Dalgleish at St George's Hospital, London.

Source

For more information on the T/Tn vaccine contact the Heather Bligh Clinic in the USA on 001 847 578 3435.

To see Professor Dalgleish, you will require an appropriate private medical referral after enquiring from your doctor about the availability of vaccines to treat your disease. Vaccine treatment cannot be used at the same time as chemotherapy.

6 Physical support therapies

The successful approach to reversing cancer and preventing it returning is always multi-modal. No single therapy, technique or substance can as yet prevail against the complexity of this disease. The exact combination of therapies and substances depends entirely on the individual patient and the skill and knowledge of the physician. This section describes useful physical therapies that can potentially help the effect of other treatments.

Hyperthermia

Background

Hyperthermia is a clinical process that has been pioneered by Professor Douwes in Germany, in which the body temperature is raised in order to help destroy cancer tumours. Research has shown that cancer cells are more sensitive to heat than normal tissues. Direct killing of cancer cells begins to occur when the cancerous tissue reaches 104-105.8°F.[63] Hyperthermia can greatly enhance the effectiveness of chemotherapy and radiotherapy.

Use

Hyperthermia is used for the treatment of cancer and may involve either increasing the temperature of the whole body or just tissue locally at the site of a cancer tumour. Heat can be localised with the use of microwave diathermy or ultrasound. Diathermy raises the body temperature by applying radio-frequency electromagnetic energy. Ultrasound causes an increase in body temperature as a result of friction produced at the molecular level when the high-energy sound waves strike the different body tissues. These procedures are particularly effective in controlling superficial tumours located on or near the skin. In whole body hyperthermia, the temperature of the whole body is taken up gradually, while the individual is sedated. This is done under extremely vigilant medical supervision. This type of treatment is often used in conjunction with low-dose chemotherapy or radiotherapy as their effect can be greatly potentiated by the heat treatment. This can therefore be a useful option for those who do not feel able or well enough to embark upon full-dose chemotherapy.

Special precautions

Patients must be strong to tolerate this therapy because enduring the high body temperatures that are induced in whole body hyperthermia is fairly unpleasant. Caution is advised with patients who have cardiovascular disease due to the extra stress that high body temperatures place upon the heart, and microwave diathermy should never be used by people with pacemakers. This therapy must always be done under expert medical supervision.

Mechanism of action

Studies have shown that hyperthermia treatment modifies cell membranes, helping to weaken them, which makes the tumour cells more susceptible to chemotherapy, radiation and immune attack

Level of evidence

Several laboratory and human studies have shown that hyperthermia can play an important role in the treatment of some cancers. At the Duke Hyperthermia Program of the Duke University Medical Centre in Durham, North Carolina, considerable success has been reported using hyperthermia to treat soft tissue sarcomas and recurrences of breast cancer.

Source and price

Hyperthermia is available in Britain at the Liongate Clinic in Tunbridge Wells, under Dr Fritz Schellander (cost available on enquiry). Telephone 01892 543535. Hyperthermia is available in Germany under its pioneer, Professor Douwes on 0049 8061 494215 (cost available on enquiry).

Detoxification

One of the most essential parts of any cancer-reversal programme is to detoxify the body at the cellular level and help promote excretion of the toxins by the liver.

The cleansing of toxins and waste products from the body helps reduce the stress on the immune system and tissue functioning generally. It is important to understand that the cause of cancer is not just the presence of a carcinogen alone, but a combination of this with the body's weakened ability to destroy cancer cells and tumours as they arise due to cellular toxicity.

There are a variety of detoxification therapies available for the intestines, liver, lymph, lungs and skin, all aimed at helping the body to eliminate toxins. There are also specific herbal remedies to help eliminate the toxic residues of both chemotherapy and radiotherapy. Detoxification also includes eliminating unwanted viruses, bacteria and parasites from the body, which may be weakening the body's ability to fight cancer, or be directly causing cancer.

Dietary detoxification

Dietary detoxification involves taking a very clean, light diet for 2-6 weeks, to allow the body to shed excessive toxins naturally. This can be done by following the 'Clean Machine' regime in the Cancer Lifeline Recipes by Jane Sen, within the Cancer Lifeline Kit. This process is ideally supported with liver herbs (see below). When this detox is finished, a healthy eating pattern should be established by following the 'Eat Right' recipes.

Herbal detoxification

Liver detoxification is required whenever overall detoxification of the body is being undertaken either as part of an anti-cancer treatment or after heavy cancer treatment. It is achieved through either coffee enemas or by taking Liver Herbs.

Coffee enemas have been shown to increase the liver's enzyme activity by up to seven times which speeds up the process of elimination of toxins from the body greatly. It is very noticeable that those using coffee enemas quickly find their skin and even the whites of their eyes becoming visibly clearer within days. Coffee enemas are performed at home by the individual.

The best way of doing this is by getting a gravity-feed enema kit from a chemist. About a pint of coffee is made from freshly ground coffee that is made half as strong as coffee that would be drunk. The other big difference from making coffee to drink is that the coffee is simmered for 10 minutes. It is then left to cool to blood temperature and filtered before putting into the enema kit. Thereafter it is run into the rectum via the nozzle provided. It is best to lie comfortably supported by pillows on one side, in bed or on a sofa covered with towels, as it necessary to attempt to hold the coffee in the rectum for around 20 minutes. Whilst in the rectum much of the coffee is absorbed straight into the portal vein, which runs directly to the liver. Once the coffee hits the liver it has a direct stimulant effect with a great enhancement on the cleansing of the blood. After the 20 minutes is up, the remaining coffee is then released into a lavatory, commode, bowl or bucket as convenient. Make sure the container is thoroughly cleansed and sterilised.

For many, the prospect of having an enema is repugnant and similar results can be observed by taking liver detox herbs. A good Liver Herbs preparation is available from Argyll Herbs at £20.45 for 450 ml.

Chest detoxification is required if the lungs have become very congested with mucus or fluid or if there is a cough that persists. Chest Herbs are also available from Argyll Herbs at £20.45 for 450 ml.

Lymph detoxification is necessary if the lymph flow has become sluggish and the tissues appear congested or 'water-logged'. Lymph Herbs are available from Argyll Herbs at £20.45 for 450 ml.

Skin detoxification is performed with lymph drainage massage or skin brushing techniques.

Chemotherapy herbs are usually made from Chinese herbs and particularly good ones are available from Anna-Maria Lavin at Kailash, in St Johns Wood, London. Telephone 0207 722 3939.

Radiation remedies are available both from homeopathy and flower remedy ranges. The homeopathic radiation remedy is called Rad Brom. This can be taken at the 200x strength on a daily basis both during, and for a week after, radiotherapy to help to antidote the effects. It can also be taken at the 30x strength in which case it will be needed about 6 hourly. The weaker 6x strength may be needed hourly. Rad Brom is available from homeopathic chemists and health food shops. The radiation flower remedy is made Galen and is available from the Bristol Cancer Help Centre shop on 0117 980 9504. Excellent radiation cream made by Louise Bradbury is also available from the Bristol shop.

Colonic irrigation

Another fairly radical form of detox is achieved by colonic irrigation. In this treatment the colon is filled with a large quantity of warm saline solution administered through the rectum. The fluid is then released and with it any debris that has adhered over time to the wall of the colon. Often surprisingly large amounts of accumulated matter are shed and it is believed that this helps the bowel to work more efficiently in its eliminatory function thereafter.

Reducing your exposure to chemicals, toxins and substances to which you are allergic

In addition to the above mentioned internal detoxification therapies, it is desirable to reduce your exposure to a variety of chemicals and toxins we commonly come into contact with. These may be in the food and water we consume, the environment in which we live and even our own homes! It is also helpful to eliminate foods and drinks from our diet to which we have an allergy. Many of us have food intolerances that are undiagnosed and which can be placing a considerable burden on the body's defences.

Cancer usually arises in areas of the body where inflammation commonly occurs. This is exactly what allergies do to us, making the tissues of our guts and lungs vulnerable. Of course this effect is most problematic when we regularly introduce strong toxins such as tobacco smoke and strong alcohol into the body. It is therefore advised that smoking is stopped altogether if you have cancer and that the consumption of alcohol is kept to an absolute minimum, being saved for special occasions only. It is helpful to have an allergy check for food and drink to which you may be allergic, so that you can eliminate these substances from the body to help reduce the immune load.

It is advisable where possible to limit your exposure of toxins in your home, where you may be exposed to toxic chemicals in many household products, cosmetics and personal care products. Although none of these products alone may present a critical toxic exposure, when many little exposures are added together they can present a cumulative toxic load that stress the body's immune system and damages cells.[64]

Many chemicals used in cosmetics and personal care products do not require full safety testing before they are allowed to be marketed and used by millions of consumers. Dr Samuel Epstein has long highlighted the potential danger of certain chemical substances in many of the personal care products that we commonly use. A useful summary can be found in 'The Safe Shoppers Bible' by Epstein & Steinman.[64] It is therefore good to attempt to use products that are known to be free of chemical carcinogens wherever possible.

Source and price

Neways International offers an extensive range of personal care, skin, hair care and household products that contain effective and safe ingredients.

The catalogue and price list detailing an extensive range of personal care, cosmetics and household products that are free from ingredients that may harm you is available from Healthy Solutions on 01454 418972.

Viral, baterial, fungal and parasite elimination

At least 15% of all cancer is currently known to be caused by viruses. For example most cancer of the cervix, many lymphomas and leukaemias and primary liver cancer are caused by viruses. These are just the cancers we know about with viral origins. We also know that stomach and oesophageal cancers can be associated with the bacteria Helicobacter Pylori. In addition to this, there are cancers that are linked with the presence of parasites in the body, which also create a source of irritation. It is strongly suspected that many more cancers will be found to have infective origins in the future. This is probably the reason why there are such high cancer rates associated with the eating of meats and animal fats as these infective agents are often passed through the animal food chain.

Infective causes of cancer must be eliminated from the body in order to stabilise your health. This will occur in part by the overall raising of immune function through healthy eating, exercise and improved mental state. However it can also be wise to take antiviral medicine such as Echinacea (mentioned earlier). Pre-cancerous cervical problems can be treated locally with a mixture of the herb Golden Seal and Tea Tree Oil in an almond oil carrier, given as a douche on a daily basis (although laser and cone biopsy are strongly recommended for CIN2 and CIN3 lesions). The presence of Helicobacter in the gut can be assessed by your doctor and, if present, be treated with antibiotics.

Parasites in the gut are traditionally treated with the herb wormwood, and Dr Gerald Green makes strong claims for the use of wormwood with an anti-candida diet for the effective treatment of cancer. Wormwood tablets are available from the Nutri-Centre at £7.49 for 100 tablets. Wormwood and Clove tablets that are also used for this purpose are available for £12.89 for 100 tablets.

However, more recently there has been a fascinating advance in complementary medicine known as complex homeopathy. In this speciality the practitioner is able to pin-point the presence of infective agents that are in the system and continuing to cause problems, often long after the acute illness they created. The agents discovered are then treated with homeopathic drops and the overall effect is to lift this infective burden from the body. This form of medicine has been pioneered by Dr Adrian Lindeman, in Devon, who has now trained a number of practitioners. Being first checked and then treated by a complex homeopath can be a very useful part of the overall jigsaw puzzle for the recovery of your health and well-being.

Three good practitioners in the UK are Janice Seeley, in Devon (01884 258143); Tim Part, in Bath (01225 329355); and Mark Salmon, in London (0207 211 3899).

Conclusion

In reading this guide, some of the remedies and treatments may have clearly seemed right for you. But this long list of possibilities may be daunting. Remember that help in putting together an integrated self-help regime can be obtained from the integrated medicine doctors listed in the Resource Directory. Or you may wish to go directly to an alternative cancer doctor or clinic to be given alternative medical treatment. It may help to know that remarkable cancer survivor Ian Gawler tried 37 forms of alternative therapy before being cured of serious secondary bone cancer! The secret of success may well be trial and error and, most important of all, to listen to your intuition and what your body is telling you.

Please let us know at Health Creation of any new discoveries you make, or of any omissions or mistakes we have made. And remember, our recommended holistic doctors and the Health Creation Mentors are here to help you via our Helpline 0845 009 3366.

We wish you every possible success with your alternative cancer treatment and would love to hear of your experiences.

All power to you in your explorations and recovery, from the Health Creation Team.

7 Resource directory

NAME/ORGANISATION	SERVICE	TELEPHONE/WEBSITE
Alternative cancer treatment suppliers		
The Nutri Centre Hale Clinic, London	Where Health Creation clients receive a 10% discount on quotation of reference ZZRMD001. The Nutri Centre also donates to the Health Creation Foundation to enable those on low incomes to obtain Health Creation Kits, Mentor Services and nutritional support at low cost.	0207 637 8436 pract@nutricentre.com
Healthy Solutions	Neways International supplier.	01454 418972
Nu-Skin UK Ltd	Pharmanex supplier.	Orders 0800 413672 Enquiries 01494 443484
Argyll Herbs	Herbal Medicines.	01984 624911
Nature's Own	Food Supplements, Vitamins and Minerals.	01684 310022
Integrated holistic cancer doctors		
Dr Rosy Daniel	Bristol. London.	0117 949 3366 0207 299 9428
Dr Roger Lichy	Hampstead, London.	0207 431 7546
Dr Sara Miller	Flax Burton, Bristol.	01275 464149

NAME/ORGANISATION	SERVICE	TELEPHONE/WEBSITE
Dr Nicola Hembry	Bristol.	0117 950 5928 info@nicolahembry.co.uk
Dr George Lewith	Southampton.	023 8033 4752
Dr Mosarif Ali	London.	0207 244 5111

Integrated medicine research and information service

Cancer Options	Cancer Options is a private, cancer consultancy where you can obtain consultancy, research and coaching for all the different cancer treatments and therapies.	0845 009 2041 www.canceroptions.co.uk

Immune therapy

Dr Julian Kenyon	Dove Clinic for Integrated Medicine Winchester, Hampshire.	01962 718000 www.doveclinic.com
Professor Gus Dalgleish	St George's Medical School, London.	0208 672 9944
Dr Thomas Nesselhut Germany	Dendritic cell therapy.	00 49 552 72056

Hyperthermia

Dr Fritz Schellander	Liongate Clinic, Tunbridge Wells.	01892 543535
Professor Douwes Germany		Fax 00 49 8061 494215

NAME/ORGANISATION	SERVICE	TELEPHONE/WEBSITE
Alternative cancer clinics and doctors UNITED KINGDOM		
Dr Fritz Schellander	Liongate Clinic, Tunbridge Wells.	01892 543535
Dr Patrick Kingsley	Leicester.	01530 223622
Dr Jan de Vries	Ayrshire.	01292 311414
Dr Rodney Adeniyi-Jones	The Regent Clinic, London.	0207 486 6354
Dr Julian Kenyon	Dove Clinic, Hampshire.	01962 718000
Dr Wendy Denning	London.	0207 224 5111
Dr Maendl (Iscador)	Anthroposophical Doctor, Bristol.	0117 949 9668
Dr Etienne Callebout	London.	0207 255 2232
Park Attwood	Anthroposophical Clinic Park Attwood clinic uses anthroposophical medicine and integrates complementary and orthodox medicine. The Clinic is designed, staffed and licensed to care for 14 in-patients and to conduct out-patient appointments. The staff consists of 6 doctors, 17 nurses and 7 therapists apart from the household and staff. Care is offered for a range of illnesses including cancer.	01299 861444 www.parkattwood.org
Lyndon Hill Clinic	Reading.	0118 940 1234

NAME/ORGANISATION	SERVICE	TELEPHONE/WEBSITE
Alternative cancer clinics and doctors INTERNATIONAL		
Professor Douwes Germany	Hyperthermia.	Fax 00 49 8061 494215
Dr Waldraut Fryda Germany	Adrenaline Therapy. By referral from Dr Schellander or Dr Daniel.	
Dr Thomas Nesselhut Germany	Dendritic cell therapy.	00 49 552 72056
Dr Michael Schachter New York, USA	Amydalin.	001 845 368 4700
Dr J Contreras Mexico	The Oasis of Hope.	011 52 664 631 61 00 www.oasisofhope.com
Dr Alexander Herzog	Klinic Benidiktus Guelle.	00 49 604 39830
Issels therapy	A holistic immunological treatment which, especially when used in conjunction with conventional treatment, can do more for people with cancer than conventional treatments according to this site.	www.issels.com

NAME/ORGANISATION	SERVICE	TELEPHONE/WEBSITE
Doctors who prescribe Carctol are:		
Dr Rosy Daniel	Bristol.	0117 9493366
	London.	0207 299 9428
Dr Mark Atkinson	London.	0207 251 2670
Dr Roger Lichy	London.	0207 431 7546
Dr Kanu Patel	Leicester.	01162 663939
Dr Prabhatsinh Chudasama	London.	0208 863 8370
Dr Milind Jani	Brighton.	01273 777448 / 01273 748600
See also http://www.newlifeayurvedicherbs.co.uk/ for further information on Carctol		

Nutritional approaches to cancer

NAME/ORGANISATION	SERVICE	TELEPHONE/WEBSITE
The Nutrition Trust Dr Chris Ashton and Dr Paul Leyman		01483 202264
Gerson Therapy UK contact Lesley Pearce		01372 817652

Alternative cancer websites

www.cancure.org

www.cancernet.nci.nih.gov

www.sph.uth.tmc.edu

www.cancerdecisions.com

www.np.edu.sg

www.howtopreventcancer.com

www.healthy.net

www.alternativemedicine.com

www.cancerguide.org

www.allabouthealth.com

www.newlifeayurvedicherbs.co.uk

www.anticancerherb.com

Further reading

Choices in Healing – Dr Michael Lerner MIT Press 1996

The Definitive Guide to Cancer, alternative treatment by John Diamond, William Lee and Burton Goldberg

Options: The Alternative Cancer Therapy Book, Richard Walters

Cancer and Its Nutritional Therapies, Dr Richard Passwater, Keats Publishing (1993)

Nutrition and Cancer: State of the Art, Positive Health, Dr Sandra Goodman (1998)

Sharks Don't Get Cancer, Dr William Lane, Avery Publishing Group (1992)

The Optimum Nutrition Bible, Patrick Holford, Piatkus (1997)

Say no to Cancer, Patrick Holford, Piatkus (1999)

Scientific information

The Research Council for Complementary Medicine
www.rccm.org.uk
0207 384 1772

The National Institute of Health, America, Office of Alternative Medicine
or the Department of Alternative Cancer Medicine, University of Houston, Texas

8 References

1   Kindles, A R, and M Radman. 'Tumour Promoter Induces Sister Chromatid Exchanges.' Proceedings of the National Academy of Sciences 75 (1978), 6149-6153.

2   Schrauzer, G N 'Selenium in Nutritional Cancer Prophylaxis: An Update.' Vitamins, Nutrition and Cancer, edited by Prosad, K N (Basel, Switzerland Karger, 1984).

3   Boik, J 'Zinc: Dietary Micronutrients and Their Effects on Cancer.' Cancer and Natural Treatment (Princeton, MN: Oregon Medical Press, 1995), 147.

4   Gershwin, M E, et al. 'The Potential Impact of Nutritional Factors on Immunological Responsiveness.' Nutrition and Immunity (Orlando, FL: Academic Press. 1985), 222.

5   Fritsche, K L and P V Johnston. 'Effect of Dietary Alpha-linolenic Acid on Growth, Metastasis, Fatty Acid Profile and Prostaglandin Production of Two Murine Mammary Adenocarcinomas.' Journal of Nutrition 120 (1990), 1601-1609.

6   Ernster L, Forsmark-Andree P: Ubiquinol: an endogenous antioxidant in aerobic organisms. Clinical investigator 72 (suppl 8): S60-S65, 1993.

7   Folkers K, Wolaniuk A: Research on coenzyme Q10 in clinical treatment and in immunomodulation. Drugs Under Experimental and Clinical Research XI (8): 539-545, 1985.

8   Folkers K, Shizukuishi S, Takemura K, et al: Increase in levels of IgG in serum of patients treated with coenzyme Q10. Research Communications in Chemical Pathology and Phamacology 38 (2): 335-338,1982.

9   Steinmetz, K A, and J D Potter. 'Vegetables, Fruit and Cancer Vol 2 Mechanisms.' Cancer Causes and Control (1991), 427-442.

10 Zhang, L and Tizard, I R, 'Activation of mouse macrophage cell line by acemannan: the major carbohydrate fraction from Aloe Vera gel'.

11 Harris, C et al 'Efficacy of acemannan in treatment of canine and feline spontaneous neoplasms', Molecular Biology 3:2, 207-213 (1991).

12 Boik, J 'Conducting research on natural agents', Cancer and Natural Medicine: A Textbook of Basic Science and Clinical Research (Princeton MN:Oregon Medical Press), 177 (1995).

13 Brown, Wood and Smith, Sodium Cyanide as a Cancer Chemotherapeutic Agent., Laboratory and Clinical Studies, American Journal Obst & Gynec, 80:907, 1960

14 Moss, R W The Cancer Industry: Unravelling the Politics (New York: Paragon House, 1989).

15 H M Chang and P P H But, eds. Pharmacology and Applications of Chinese Materia Medica (Singapore: World Scientific,1987), 1041-6.

16 K S Zhao et al., 'Enhancement of the Immune Response in Mice by Astragalus membranaceus', Immunopharmacol 20 (1988): 225-33.

17 Boik, J Anti-tumour and anticancer effects of botanical agents. Cancer & Natural Medicine: A Textbook of Basic Science and Clinical Research. Princeton, Minnesota: Oregon Medical Press Publishers; 1996; 120-8.

18 Chu, D T Wong, W and Mavligit, g, (1998), Immunotherapy with Chinese medicinal herbs. 11. Reversal of cyclophosphamide-induced immune suppression by administration of fractionated Astralagus membranaceous in vivo. Journal of Clinical and Laboratory Immunology 25:125-129.

19 U S Patent No. 4,844,901. Oxindole alkaloids, from una de gato (Cat's Claw), have immune-stimulating properties.

20 Melchart, D, Linde, K., Worku, F et al (1994) Immunomodulation with Echinacea – a systematic review of controlled clinical trials. Phytomedicine 1:245-254

21 Erhard, M. et al, 'Effects of Echinacea, Aconium, Lachesis and Apis extractsand their combinations on phagocytosis of human granulocytes', Phytother Res, vol 8 pp14-17 (1994).

22 Moss, R 'Essiac' Cancer Therapy: The Independent Consumer's Guide (New York; Equinox Press, 1992), 146-147. Moss reviews the technical cancer-related research on Essiac; many substances isolated from herbs in Essiac show specific kinds of anticancer activity.

23 Chen Q H et al 'Studies on Chinese Rhubarb XII. Effect of Anthraquinone Derivatives on the Respiration and Glycolysis of Ehrlich Ascites Carcinoma Cells.' Acta Pharmaceutica Sinica 15 (1980), 65-70.

24 Lu, M, and Q H Chen 'Biochemical Study of Chinese Rhubarb XXIX. Inhibitory Effects of Anthraquinone Derivatives on P338 Leukaemia in Mice.' Journal of China Pharmacology University 20 (1989), 155-157.

25 Morita, K et al 'A Desmutagenic Factor Isolated from Burdock.' Mutation Research 129 (1984), 25-31.

26 Cyong, J C et al, J Ethno Pharmacol, vol 19, 279-83 (1987).

27 Pinto, J T, Qiao, C H, Xing, J, Rivlin, R S, Protomastro, M L, Weissler, M L and Heston, W D W, 1999. 'Effects of garlic thioallylic derivatives on growth, glutathione concentration, and polyamine formation of human prostate carcinoma cells in culture.' Am. J Clin. Nutr. See also: Li, G, Qiao, C H, Lin, R I, Pinto, J, Osborne, M P and Tiwari, R K, 1995. Antiproliferative effects of garlic constituents in cultured human breast cancer cells. Oncology Rpts,2, 787-791.

28 Lau, B H S et al 'Allium sativum (Garlic) and Cancer Prevention.' Nutrition Research 10 (1990), 937-948.

29 Lin, R S Garlic and Health: Recent Advances in Research (Irvine, CA: International Academy of Health and Fitness, 1994), 23.

30 Chisaka, T et al Chemical and Pharmaceutical Bulletin (1988). Cited in: Wilner, J 'Green Tea.' The Cancer Solution (Boca Raton, FL: Peltec Publishing, 1994), 75.

31 Bu-Abbas, A et al 'Marked Antimutagenic Potential of Aqueous Green Tea Extracts: Mechanism of Action.' Mutagenesis 9 (1994), 325-331.

32 A. Mukhtar, H et al 'Green Tea and Skin – Anticarcinogenic Effects.' Journal of Investigative Dermatology 102 (1994), 3-7.

33 Klaunig, J E 'Chemopreventative Effects of Green Tea Components on Hepatic Carcinogenesis.' Preventative Medicine 21 (1992), 510-519. See also: Gao, Y T et al, 'Reduced Risk of Esophageal Cancer associated with Green Tea Consumption.' Journal of the National Cancer Institute 86 (1994), 855-858.

34 Michnoviez, J J, Bradlow, H L, 'Altered estrogen metabolism and excretion in humans following consumption of indole-3-carbinol'. Nutr Cancer. 1991;16(1): 59-66.

35 Dosage range study of Indole-3-carbinol in breast cancer prevention. J Cell Biochem Supplement 1997. 28-29: 111-6.

36 Cover CM et al. 'Indole-3-carbinol and tamoxifen co-operate to arrest the cell cycle of MCF7 Human Breast Cancer Cells'. Cancer Research. 1999; 59; 1244-1251.

37 Kiene, H 'Clinical Studies on Mistletoe Therapy for Cancerous Diseases: A Review.' Therapeutikon 3:6 (1989), 347-350.

38 Hajito, T, and C Lanzerein. 'Natural Killer and Antibody-Department Cell-mediated Cytotoxity and Large Granular Lymphocyte Frequencies in Viscum album-Treated Breast

Cancer Patients.' Oncology Suppl 1 (1986), 93-97. See also: Hajito, T 'Immunomodulatory Effects of Iscador: A Viscum album Preparation.' Oncology 43 Suppl 1 (1986), 51-65.

39 Nienhaus, J 'Tumour Inhibition and Thymus Stimulation with Mistletoe Preparations.' Elemente Naturowissenschaft 13 (1970), 45-54.

40 Adachi, K et al 'Potentiation of Host-mediated Antitumour Activity in Mice by Beta-glucan Obtained from Grifola frondosa (Maitake). 'Chemical & Pharmacological Bulletin 35:1 (1987), 262-270.

41 Matsuoka, H, Yano, K, Seo, Y, et al 'Usefulness of lymphocyte subset change as an indicator for predicting survival time and effectiveness of treatment with the immunopotentiator lentinan' Anticancer Research 1995; 15:2291-96.

42 Hirazumi, A, Furusawa, E, 'Immunomodulation Contributes to the Anticancer Activity of Morinda Citrifolia (Noni) Fruit Juice' Proc.West. Pharmacol. Soc. 39 (1996) 7-9.

43 Hirazumi, A., Furusawa, E 'An Immunomodulatory Polysaccharide-Rich Substance from the Fruit Juice of Morinda Citrifolia (Noni) with Antitumour Activity', Department of Pharmacology, John A Burns School of Medicine, Hawaii, HI 96822 USA. Phytotherapy Research 1999 Aug;13(5):380-7.

44 Hirazumi,A, Furusawa, E, 'Anticancer Activity of Morinda Citrifolia (Noni) on Intraperitoneally Implanted Lewis Lung Carcinoma in Syngenic Mice.' Proc West Pharmacol Soc 1994;37:145-6.

45 Rao, K V 'Quinone Natural Products. Streptonigrin (NSC-45383) and Lapachol (NSC-11905) Structure-activity Relationships.' Cancer Chemotherapy Reports (Part 2) 4:4 (1974), 11-17.

46 Santana, C F et al 'Preliminary Observations with the Use of Lapachol in Human Patients Bearing Malignant Neoplasms.' Revista de Instituto de Antibioticos 20 (1980/1981), 61-68. Cited in: Werbach, M R, and M T Murray, Botanical Influences on Illness (Tarzana, CA: Third Line Press, 1994).

47 Linardi, M D C et al 'A Lapachol Derivative Active against Mouse Lymphocyte Leukemia P- 388.' Journal of Medicinal Chemistry 18:11 (1975), 1159-1162.

48 Small, E J, Frohlich, M.W., Bok, R., Shinohara, K et al 'Prospective trial of the herbal supplement PC-Specs in patients with progressive prostate cancer.' Journal of Clinical Oncology 18(21): 3595-3603 (2000).

49 Nagabhushan, M, and S.V. Bhide. 'Curcumin as an Inhibitor of Cancer.' Journal of the American College of Nutrition 11:2 (1992). 192-198.

50 Rao, C V et al 'Chemoprevention of Colon Carcinogenesis by Dietary Curcumin, a Naturally Occurring Plant Phenolic Compound.' Cancer Research 55:2 (1995), 259-266.

51 Polasa, K et al 'Effect of Turmeric on Urinary Mutagens in Smokers.' Mutagen 7:2 (1992), 107-109.

52 Nagabhushan, M, and S V Bhide 'Curcumin as an Inhibitor of Cancer.' Journal of the American College of Nutrition 11:2 (1992). 192-198.

53   Chang, K J, Lee T T Y, Linares-Cruz, G. 'Influences of percutaneous administration of estradiol on human breast epithelial cell cycle in vivo'. Journal of Fertility and Sterility 1995; 63; 7865-7891.

54   Oikawa, T et al 'A Novel Angiogenic Inhibitor Derived from Japanese Shark Cartilage. Extraction and estimation of inhibitory activities toward tumour and embryonic angiogenesis.' Cancer Letters 52 (1990), 181-186

55   Gold, J 'Hydrazine Sulphate: A Current Perspective.' Nutrition and Cancer 9:2-3 (1987), 59-66.

56   Filov, V A et al 'Results of Clinical Evaluation of Hydrazine Sulphate.' Voprosy Onkologii 36:6 (1990), 721-726. See also: Gershanovich, M.L. et al. 'Results of Clinical Study of Antitumour Action of Hydrazine Sulphate.' Nutrition and Cancer 3 (1981), 7-12.

57   Pelton, Ross and Lee, Overholser. Alternatives in Cancer Therapy (New York: Fireside/Simon & Schuster, 1994), Chapter 20, Footnote 5. Tumour cell surfaces contain large amounts of surfactants (glycoproteins and other large molecular surface-active agents), which have hydrophobic and hydrophilic properties at nonpolar sites, respectively, producing a structured water matrix surrounding cancer cells that is markedly different from that surrounding normal cells.

58   Pelton, Ross and Lee Overholser. Alternatives in Cancer Therapy (New York: Fireside/Simon & Schuster, 1994), Chapter 20, Footnote 1.

59 Danopoulus, E D, et al ' Eleven Years of Oral /urea Treatment in Liver Malignancies.' Clinical Oncology 7 (1981), 281-289.

60 Clement, R J et al 'Peritoneal Mesothelioma' Quantum Treatment 1 (1988), 68-73.

61 Springer, G F 'T and Tn General Carcinoma Autoantigens.' Science 224 (1984), 1198-1206.

62 Springer, G F 'T/Tn Antigen: Two Decades of Experience in Early Immuno-Detection and Therapy of Human Carcinoma.' Jung Foundation Proceedings (Stuttgart, Germany: G. Thieme) in press.

63 Dewhirst, M, Professor of Radiation Oncology and Director of the Duke Hyperthermia Program at the Duke University Medical Centre, Durham, North Carolina, Personal Communications (1996).

64 Steinman, D, and S S Epstein. The Safe Shopper's Bible (New York:Macmillan, 1994).